Leadership and Management Core Competencies

Guest Editors

MICHAEL HOUSTON, MD
BARRY D. SARVET, MD

CHILD AND ADOLESCENT PSYCHIATRIC CLINICS OF NORTH AMERICA

www.childpsych.theclinics.com

Consulting Editor
HARSH K. TRIVEDI, MD

January 2010 • Volume 19 • Number 1

SAUNDERS an imprint of ELSEVIER, Inc.

W.B. SAUNDERS COMPANY

A Division of Elsevier Inc.

Elsevier Inc. ● 1600 John F. Kennedy Boulevard ● Suite 1800 ● Philadelphia, Pennsylvania 19103-2899

http://www.childpsych.theclinics.com

CHILD AND ADOLESCENT PSYCHIATRIC CLINICS OF NORTH AMERICA Volume 19, Number 1
January 2010 ISSN 1056–4993, ISBN-13: 978-1-4377-1802-7

Editor: Sarah E. Barth
Developmental Editor: Donald Mumford

Child and Adolescent Psychiatric Clinics of North America (ISSN 1056-4993) is published quarterly by Elsevier Inc., 360 Park Avenue South, New York, NY 10010-1710. Months of issue are January, April, July, and October. Business and Editorial Offices: 1600 John F. Kennedy Boulevard, Suite 1800, Philadelphia, PA 19103-2899. Periodicals postage paid at New York, NY and additional mailing offices. Subscription prices are $257.00 per year (US individuals), $386.00 per year (US institutions), $132.00 per year (US students), $292.00 per year (Canadian individuals), $466.00 per year (Canadian institutions), $168.00 per year (Canadian students), $347.00 per year (international individuals), $466.00 per year (international institutions), and $168.00 per year (international students). International air speed delivery is included in all Clinics subscription prices. All prices are subject to change without notice. **POSTMASTER:** Send address changes to Child and Adolescent Psychiatric Clinics of North America, Elsevier Health Sciences Division, Subscription Customer Service, 3251 Riverport Lane, Maryland Heights, MO 63043. **Customer Service: 1-800-654-2452 (U.S. and Canada); 314-447-8871 (outside U.S. and Canada). Fax: 314-447-8029. E-mail: JournalsCustomerService-usa@ elsevier.com (for print support) or journalsonlinesupport-usa@elsevier.com (for online support).**

Reprints. For copies of 100 or more of articles in this publication, please contact the Commercial Reprints Department, Elsevier Inc., 360 Park Avenue South, New York, New York 10010-1710 Tel.: (212) 633-3812; Fax: (212) 462-1935, e-mail: reprints@elsevier.com.

Child and Adolescent Psychiatric Clinics of North America is covered in *MEDLINE/PubMed (Index Medicus), ISI, SSCI, Research Alert, Social Search, Current Contents,* and *EMBASE/Excerpta Medica.*

Printed and bound by CPI Group (UK) Ltd, Croydon, CR0 4YY

Transferred to Digital Print 2011

Contributors

CONSULTING EDITOR

HARSH K. TRIVEDI, MD
Site Training Director and Director of Adolescent Services, E.P. Bradley Hospital; Assistant Professor of Psychiatry and Human Behavior (Clinical), Brown Medical School; President, Rhode Island Council for Child and Adolescent Psychiatry, East Providence, Rhode Island

CONSULTING EDITOR EMERITUS

ANDRÉS MARTIN, MD, MPH

FOUNDING CONSULTING EDITOR

MELVIN LEWIS, MBBS, FRCPSYCH, DCH

GUEST EDITORS

MICHAEL HOUSTON, MD
Associate Clinical Professor of Psychiatry, Department of Psychiatry and Behavioral Sciences; Assistant Clinical Professor of Pediatrics, Department of Pediatrics, George Washington University Medical School, Washington, District of Columbia

BARRY D. SARVET, MD
Chief, Division of Child and Adolescent Psychiatry, Baystate Medical Center, Clinical Associate Professor, Tufts University School of Medicine, Springfield, Massachusetts

AUTHORS

STEVEN ADELSHEIM, MD
Professor of Psychiatry, Pediatrics and Family and Community Medicine and Director of Center for Rural and Community Behavioral Health, University of New Mexico, Albuquerque, New Mexico

SHERRY BARRON-SEABROOK, MD
Associate Professor in Psychiatry, Columbia University, College of Physicians and Surgeons, New York, New York

CHRISTOPHER BELLONCI, MD
Medical Director and Senior Clinical Consultant, Walker, Needham, Massachusetts

DAVID BERLAND, MD
Department of Psychiatry, St Louis University School of Medicine, St Louis, Missouri

SHIRAZ BUTT, MD
Assistant Professor of Psychiatry, Rush University Medical Center, Chicago; Medical Director, Maryville Academy, Des Plaines, Illinois

MARK CHENVEN, MD
Associate Clinical Professor, Division of Child and Adolescent Psychiatry, Department of Psychiatry, UCSD Medical School; Sr. Vice President, Clinical Operations, Vista Hill Foundation, San Diego, California; Co-Chair, Work Group on Community Systems of Care, American Academy of Child & Adolescent Psychiatry

MARTIN GLASSER, MD
Medical Director, Behavioral Health, Anthem Blue Cross National Accounts, San Diego, California

MICHAEL HOUSTON, MD
Associate Clinical Professor of Psychiatry, Department of Psychiatry and Behavioral Sciences; Assistant Clinical Professor of Pediatrics, Department of Pediatrics, George Washington University Medical School, Washington, District of Columbia

ROBERT L. KLAEHN, MD
Medical Director, Arizona Division of Developmental Disabilities, Arizona Department of Economic Security, Phoenix, Arizona; Faculty, Maricopa Integrated Health System Child Psychiatry Residency Program, Phoenix, Arizona

AVRON KRIECHMAN, MD
Assistant Professor of Psychiatry, Child, Adolescent and Family Psychiatrist and Telehealth Specialist, Department of Psychiatry, Center for Rural and Community Behavioral Health, University of New Mexico, Albuquerque, New Mexico

ERIN MALLOY, MD
Associate Professor and Director, Child and Adolescent Inpatient Services, Department of Psychiatry, University of North Carolina, Chapel Hill, North Carolina

MICHAEL W. NAYLOR, MD
Clinical Psychiatry, Department of Psychiatry, University of Illinois; Director, Division of Child and Adolescent Psychiatry; and Director, Behavioral Health and Welfare Program, Institute for Juvenile Research, Chicago, Illinois

KRISTIN KROEGER PTAKOWSKI, BA
Senior Deputy Executive Director, Director of Government Affairs & Clinical Practice, American Academy of Child and Adolescent Psychiatry, Washington, District of Columbia

MELINA SALVADOR, MA
Associate Research Scientist, Department of Psychiatry, Center for Rural and Community Behavioral Health, University of New Mexico, Albuquerque, New Mexico

BARRY D. SARVET, MD
Chief, Division of Child and Adolescent Psychiatry, Baystate Medical Center, Clinical Associate Professor, Tufts University School of Medicine, Springfield, Massachusetts

ROBERT K. SCHRETER, MD
Clinical Associate Professor of Psychiatry, University of Maryland School of Medicine, and Clinical Assistant Professor of Psychiatry, Johns Hopkins School of Medicine, Lutherville, Maryland

SANDRA B. SEXSON, MD
Professor, Psychiatry and Pediatrics, Chief, Division of Child, Adolescent and Family
Psychiatry, and Director of Training, in Child and Adolescent Psychiatry, Department
of Psychiatry and Health Behavior, Medical College of Georgia, Augusta, Georgia

BENJAMIN SHAIN, MD, PhD
Head, Division of Child and Adolescent Psychiatry, Northshore University HealthSystem,
Highland Park; Clinical Assistant Professor, University of Chicago, Chicago, Illinois

ADRIAN SONDHEIMER, MD
Formerly Associate Professor of Psychiatry and Research Teaching Specialist,
Division of Child and Adolescent Psychiatry, UMDNJ-New Jersey Medical School,
Newark, New Jersey

MICHAEL SORTER, MD
Associate Professor and Director, Division of Child and Adolescent Psychiatry, Cincinnati
Children's Hospital Medical Center, University of Cincinnati, Cincinnati, Ohio

LYNN WEGNER, MD, FAAP
Chief, Division of Developmental and Behavioral Pediatrics, University of North Carolina
School of Medicine, Chapel Hill, North Carolina

ALBERT A. ZACHIK, MD
Director, Department of Health and Mental Hygiene, Office of Child and Adolescent
Services, State of Maryland Mental Hygiene Administration, Spring Grove Hospital
Center, Catonsville, Maryland

Cover artwork courtesy of Socorro Rivera G., Mexico City, Mexico

Contents

> Inpatient child and adolescent psychiatry leadership roles are often multi-
> faceted, necessitating strong clinical knowledge and skills, organizational
> and leadership abilities, and in the academic setting the desire and skill in
> teaching and research. Early career psychiatrists who do possess these at-
> tributes may find themselves unprepared for such challenges as dealing
> with complex administrative and economic issues, accreditation, legal mat-
> ters, and multitasking. This article offers a primer addressing these basic is-
> sues and in managing change through quality improvement processes.

> Many different programs define themselves or are defined as residential
> treatment centers (RTCs). These range from small, freestanding, private,
> nonprofit programs to subacute units within large, for-profit health care
> systems. This article focuses on the role of the physician leader in commu-
> nity-based, nonmedical institutions. First, the physician's role in an RTC is
> to optimize clinical outcomes through direct service, teaching, training,
> coaching, and consulting with the child and family and the child care, mul-
> tidisciplinary, educational, and administrative staff. Physician leaders are
> needed to integrate and translate the various assessments of the child's
> needs and strengths into a coherent narrative that can be used for treat-
> ment planning within the RTC and in the child's home and community.
> Second, physician leadership can help ensure that programs remain fam-
> ily-centered and that they use the best available evidence-based prac-
> tices. Third, physician leaders must help the RTC to develop and sustain
> its unifying theory of treatment and to use this theory to guide its practice,
> mission, and vision. Physician leaders in RTC must be "trilingual and tricul-
> tural" and adept in the mental health, special education, and child welfare
> systems to be effective advocates for youth and their families.

> Directing child and adolescent psychiatry (CAP) training for residents is
> a complex and challenging administrative task that encompasses the

broad creativity of the orchestral conductor, the social and interpersonal effectiveness of the best politician, and the orientation to details of the finest accountant. This article examines these roles in detail, recognizing the leadership, administrative, and managerial achievements of the successful child and adolescent program director. Resources for optimizing the chances for success in each of these areas, and the common pitfalls to avoid, are identified and discussed. The article concludes with suggestions for CAP training directors to influence medical student education. Although challenging and sometimes frustrating, the role of the program director in CAP training is almost always exciting and rewarding.

Child and adolescent psychiatrists are in a unique position to provide administrative and clinical leadership to public agencies. In mental health, services for children and adolescents in early childhood, school, child welfare, and juvenile justice settings, transition-aged youth programs, workforce development, family and youth leadership programs, and use of Medicaid waivers for home- and community-based service system development are described. In child welfare, collaboration between an academic child psychiatry department and a state child welfare department is described. In developmental disabilities, the role of the child and adolescent psychiatrist administrator is described providing administrative leadership, clinical consultation, quality review, and oversight of health and behavioral health plans for persons with developmental disabilities.

The child and adolescent psychiatrist cannot practice in today's world without interacting with the world of insurance and managed care. This article reviews the history of the development of the managed care industry. It also examines the variety of roles clinicians play, whether as members of physician networks, as a peer or utilization reviewers, or as medical directors. The skills required of the physician employee and the contractual and ethical concerns are discussed.

Part II: Management Core Competencies for Child and Adolescent Psychiatrists

The manager of a psychiatric practice must create and direct a clinical delivery system, design and oversee the administrative services necessary to support the system, and guide the business operations that contribute to its success. Regardless of the size of the practice, the psychiatrist administrator must handle seven core administrative responsibilities and oversee individual functions and capabilities within each domain. These responsibilities include practice development, clinical services management, medical office operations, clinical management, information management, business management, and risk management. This article provides a road-map for creating and sustaining successful clinical and administrative endeavors. It can also be used by existing practices as an audit instrument to provide a snapshot of current capabilities so that strengths as well as opportunities for continued growth can be identified.

Since the early 1990s, Current Procedure Terminology (CPT) has been the gold standard for billing for medical services. After reviewing the historical context of CPT coding, this article presents the coding methodology, discussion of specialty codes (psychiatric and other specialty codes of potential use to child and adolescent psychiatrists), and the evaluation and management (E/M) codes. Various coding options for common clinical encounters are also presented.

This article addresses the practical and legal issues related to the psychiatric medical record, with an emphasis on the issues related to confidentiality. Implications of HIPAA (Health Insurance Portability and Accountability Act) legislation for the practice of child and adolescent psychiatry are addressed. The advantages and disadvantages of electronic medical records are reviewed, with guidelines for selecting software for solo and group practices.

This article examines ethics (the philosophic study of "doing the right thing") and risk management (the practice that seeks to manage the likelihood of "doing the wrong thing") and the relationship between them in the context of administrative child and adolescent psychiatry. Issues that affect child and adolescent psychiatrists who manage staff and business units and clinical practitioners who treat and manage individual patients are addressed. Malpractice, budgeting, credentialing, boundaries, assessment, documentation, treatment, research, dangerousness, and confidentiality are among the topics reviewed.

The mental health community has made tremendous strides in eradicating stigma, demanding policy change, and improving the lives of children and adolescents with mental illnesses, accomplished through advocacy at all government levels and assisted by community involvement. However, addressing access to care for children and adolescents with mental illnesses is still challenging. Legislators are often unaware of children's mental health issues. Advocacy includes working directly with legislators and policy makers, working with a school's administration to meet the unique needs of the child, appealing against the managed care company's denial of specific treatment or formulary approval, and educating and collaborating with primary care physicians. Three principles need to be understood: change takes time, persistence is absolute, and compromise is inevitable.

Part III: Emerging Service Delivery Models

By working in collaboration with pediatric primary care providers, child and adolescent psychiatrists have the opportunity to address significant levels of unmet need for the majority of children and teenagers with serious mental health problems who have been unable to gain access to care. Effective collaboration with primary care represents a significant change from practice-as-usual for many child and adolescent psychiatrists. Implementation of progressive levels of collaborative practice, from the improvement of provider communication through the development of comprehensive collaborative systems, may be possible with sustained management efforts and application of process improvement methodology.

Because the majority of children with mental health needs are most likely to receive treatment in a school setting, there is a long history of linking child and adolescent psychiatrists to schools. Psychiatrists traditionally have been involved in assessing, diagnosing, and treating the severely mentally ill or consulting with school-based providers. With no end in sight to the dearth of child and adolescent psychiatrists, not to mention child and adolescent behavioral health providers in other disciplines, this role has been broadened in recent years by several programs in which the child and adolescent psychiatrist provides flexible, population-based, systemic, and context-specific approaches to working in schools. In this article, the authors first review some of the traditional roles for child and adolescent psychiatrists working in school mental health settings. Then 2 national programs are highlighted, which successfully integrate psychiatrist trainees into comprehensive school mental health programs. The theoretical approach to a specific community-oriented, strengths-based model for school mental health support used in New Mexico by the University of New Mexico (UNM) Psychiatry Department's Center for Rural and Community Behavioral Health school telepsychiatry program, which supports rural and frontier school mental health programs and school-based health centers, is discussed in detail. The UNM model involves a strength-and resiliency-based collaboration between the child and adolescent psychiatrist, students, families, educators, and those who support them. The psychiatrist co-creates a "community of concern" and support for students, including not only customary participants such as parents, educators, and health care providers but also peers, families of choice, lay professionals, community gatekeepers, and others identified by the student as critical to his or her well-being. The advantages for child and adolescent psychiatry trainees being exposed to a wider variety of potential roles working with schools are also discussed.

Although the future of the systems of care model continues to evolve, the core values of child psychiatry are well supported and well served in this emerging arena of public children's mental health service delivery. A substantial body of evidence supports the concepts and practices of family-driven care congruent with wraparound principles and practices. Individual and system outcomes data show efficacy for programs that integrate traditional professional services with consumer-centric wraparound approaches, such as mentoring, team decision making, and community-based services and supports. Integrative interagency practice, fostering cross-agency collaboration to address the needs of at-risk populations, has been shown to be central in providing supports for families and youth.

FORTHCOMING ISSUES

RECENT ISSUES

THE CLINICS ARE NOW AVAILABLE ONLINE!

Access your subscription at:
www.theclinics.com

Foreword
All those things they didn't teach me in medical school...

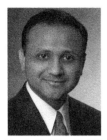

Harsh K. Trivedi, MD
Consulting Editor

Before anything else, preparation is the key to success.
                                        —*Alexander Graham Bell*

Through the entirety of medical training, there is a fundamental notion that you are putting together the building blocks of your medical career. There is a steadfast belief that the hours of diligent study and clinical training are preparing you for your professional career to come. Little do most of us realize, until after completing training, that there is another completely different education that would also have been quite helpful. Learning how to conduct a patient interview, knowing how to differentially diagnose illnesses, and developing skills to better treat patients are but a part of this education.

This is more evident when you are staring at the CPT codes in front of you (and aren't exactly sure whether to code a 90802, 90801+90802, 90801+90807/13, 90801+90807/13+90864/47, 99205, or 99245 for your initial evaluation visits). You start to feel like it wouldn't have hurt to learn a few more things in training. A short while later, when it becomes your issue to redirect the behavior of a passive-aggressive staff member, you wish someone had helped you expand your skill set to add a few more building blocks along the way. If you are then lucky enough to be propelled into a management role, when you now sit across the table from that staff member to tell them that their employment is being terminated, you really do wish that someone had shown you how to do it and to do it well. Although these caricatures of possible scenarios are provided to illustrate a point, the reality is that many of us are faced with similar situations daily in our medical careers. Most of us were never taught how to do these things nor did we receive any formal schooling on leadership or management.

This issue is an earnest attempt to put together a practical primer on developing these very necessary skills. I thank Michael Houston and Barry Sarvet for agreeing

Child Adolesc Psychiatric Clin N Am 19 (2010) xiii–xiv
doi:10.1016/j.chc.2009.09.003   **childpsych.theclinics.com**
1056-4993/09/$ – see front matter © 2010 Elsevier Inc. All rights reserved.

to guest edit this issue. Their ability to organize a structure which makes meaning of these topics is much appreciated. Many things discussed within these pages are often thought of as "on the job training" or "things that you just pick up along the way." As many of us already know, although trial by fire does eventually get you there, there are often less painful and less nerve-racking methods as well. The wonderful contributors to this issue are all leaders in the field and I thank them for sharing their expertise.

Lastly, my 'formal' education on this topic came from joining the Healthcare Access and Economics Committee of the American Academy of Child and Adolescent Psychiatry. A number of the contributors are also members of this group. Having had the good fortune of learning from them since the time I was in training and recently having the honor to be named as a co-chair, this has been one of the most valuable experiences in my professional career. I offer you this issue as my attempt to share their wisdom, and that of other leaders in the field, with you.

Harsh K. Trivedi, MD
Site Training Director and Director of Adolescent Services
E.P. Bradley Hospital
Assistant Professor of Psychiatry and Human Behavior (Clinical)
Brown Medical School
President, Rhode Island Council for Child and Adolescent Psychiatry
East Providence, RI 02915, USA

E-mail address:
harsh_trivedi@brown.edu

Preface
Leadership and Management
Core Competencies

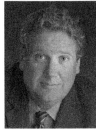 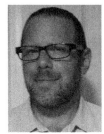

Michael Houston, MD   Barry D. Sarvet, MD
Guest Editors

Management is doing things right; leadership is doing the right things.
—*Peter F. Drucker*

Much of the medical literature in child and adolescent psychiatry is correctly focused on the nature of the illnesses that afflict our patients and the technical aspects of their treatment. Yet, in the real world within which we all work and practice following residency, our patients rely on well-functioning systems for the delivery of our services. These systems do not run themselves, and for optimal functioning, require the involvement of child and adolescent psychiatrists with substantial leadership and management skills, as well as a thorough understanding of the business and management of health care services. Indeed, it is often these areas that produce the greatest anxiety for not only the newly graduated child and adolescent psychiatrist, but also the more senior physician promoted to a leadership position as a reward for clinical, scientific, or educational achievements. Not unlike our clinical knowledge base, the skills necessary to be an effective leader and administrator are constantly evolving both in substance and complexity. This is true whether one works as a leader of a clinical service team, a medical director of a clinic or inpatient unit, a training director, a solo practitioner, or any of a variety of administrative roles for physicians in either the public or the private sector of our health care system.

As child and adolescent psychiatrists, we are fortunate that our clinical training, first as residents in general psychiatry and then as child "fellows," serves as a solid foundation for moving into leadership roles. Team management skills, regardless of whether they are explicitly taught, are part of most residents' inpatient experiences. Group and family processes, systems theory in community psychiatry, the development of sophisticated communication skills and empathic listening, and the fundamental concepts of transference and countertransference are ordinarily a part

Child Adolesc Psychiatric Clin N Am 19 (2010) xv–xvii
doi:10.1016/j.chc.2009.09.002   **childpsych.theclinics.com**

of residency training in psychiatry and also provide important lessons regarding managing people and facilitating effective work groups. These fundamental skills, along with a natural interest in making a difference in the lives of larger numbers of children and adolescents than can be seen by an individual clinician, often lead child and adolescent psychiatrists to gravitate toward leadership roles.

The articles in the first section of this issue are focused on outlining the skill set and knowledge base the physician leader will use in a variety of common practice settings. Beginning with a focus on inpatient leadership where many newly graduated clinicians find themselves working, Malloy, Butt, and Sorter outline the basics of staff and program development and walk through several case examples highlighting the multiple levels of complexity that an inpatient medical director will encounter. Appropriately they include a subsection on the theory and practice of quality improvement that is integral to the ongoing success of any effective clinical program. In Bellonci's article, a compelling model of medical leadership in the residential treatment center level of care is described, with an emphasis on facilitating effective multidisciplinary work and strength-based program design. Sexson's article on the role of the training director in child and adolescent psychiatry provides a unique primer for those new to this role, and highlights both the profound challenges, responsibilities, and rewards of this position. The public sector offers a vast array of opportunities for an effective leader to dramatically shape the care of our most vulnerable patients. Zachik, Naylor, and Klaehn have used their combined experience working within different areas of the public system to illustrate three different approaches to leadership within complex systems of care. The section on physician leadership closes with Glasser's fascinating article reviewing the history of the managed care industry and the ways in which physician leaders may work within this sector of the health care system to improve mental health treatment for children and adolescents.

The second section of this issue, focusing more specifically on discrete management topics, starts off with Schreter's engaging article on practice management that provides one of the most thorough overviews of the launching of a solo or group practice from scratch. Additional articles focus on insurance reimbursement and the complexities of coding (Berland, Shain, and Barron-Seabrook) and the issues involved in record keeping and HIPAA regulations (Houston). Sondhiemer's article on ethics and risk management should be read by clinicians at any stage in their careers, as he breaks these complicated topics down in a manner that allows one to integrate the necessary principles into one's day-to-day practice. The final piece of this section, Kroeger Ptakowski's article on advocacy for child and adolescent psychiatrists, provides both an inspirational and practical message for the members of our profession regarding the profound impact of government and legislation on children's mental health services, and the importance of getting involved in the legislative process.

The final section of the issue is focused on emerging service delivery models. The extreme and ongoing shortage of mental health professionals, and specifically child and adolescent psychiatrists, require that we look beyond the typical solo and group practice settings if, as a profession, we will ever address the mental health needs of our nation's children. Although by no means exhaustive, we chose three specific areas to illustrate the ways in which well-planned and well-implemented models can improve access to care. Sarvet and Wegner provide an overview of approaches for pediatricians and child and adolescent psychiatrists to build effective collaborative practices, thereby meeting treatment needs in the familiar setting of the child's medical home. Although school-based mental health programs are by no means new, Kriechman, Salvador, and Adelsheim have contributed an article that outlines the fundamental attributes of effective school-based programs that are flexible enough to serve the needs of diverse communities. Last, we include an article written by Chenven that highlights the utility and complexity of community-based systems of care, an often overlooked but integral part of our nation's mental health care delivery system for the most vulnerable segments of the population.

The *Child and Adolescent Psychiatry Clinics* last addressed administrative psychiatry in January of 2002 in an issue edited by Schowalter.[1] Some of the topics addressed here will be familiar to the readers of that issue. Our hope was to not only provide an updated perspective on some of the topics explored by Schowalter and colleagues, but also to focus on the leadership skills and elements of effective management that are a necessary part of the knowledge base of the practicing child and adolescent psychiatrist in the variety of settings in which we practice. We are honored to have been asked to serve as guest editors and wish to thank Dr Harsh Trivedi, Consulting Editor of the *Child and Adolescent Psychiatric Clinics of North America* for providing this opportunity. We also wish to express our appreciation to all the contributors to this issue whose collective wisdom and experience made this a rewarding experience. This issue would not be possible without the direction, support, and encouragement of Sarah Barth at Elsevier, whose professionalism and understanding is an example of effective leadership to us all.

Michael Houston, MD
Department of Psychiatry and Behavioral Sciences
George Washington University Medical School
Washington, DC, USA
Department of Pediatrics
George Washington University Medical School
2150 Pennsylvania Ave., NW, 8th Floor
Washington, DC 20037, USA

Barry D. Sarvet, MD
Division of Child and Adolescent Psychiatry
Baystate Medical Center
Tufts University School of Medicine
3300 Main Street, 4th Floor
Springfield, MA 01199, USA

E-mail addresses:
mhoustonmd@gmail.com (M. Houston)
barry.sarvet@bhs.org (B.D. Sarvet)

REFERENCE

1. Schowalter J, editor. Administrative psychiatry. Child Adolesc Psychiatr Clin N Am 2002;11(1).

Physician Leadership and Quality Improvement in the Acute Child and Adolescent Psychiatric Care Setting

Erin Malloy, MD[a],*, Shiraz Butt, MD[b,d], Michael Sorter, MD[c]

KEYWORDS

- Inpatient • Psychiatry • Leadership • Administration
- Child • Adolescent

Early career child and adolescent psychiatrists report feeling inadequately trained in the areas of leadership and administrative skills, business management, and health care economics.[1] Although child and adolescent psychiatric training programs provide residents with a significant amount of clinical experience in inpatient settings, emphasis is largely on providing clinical care. Furthermore, exposure to inpatient care is often provided in academic or state hospital settings. Early career child and adolescent psychiatrists who take on leadership roles in acute inpatient settings may find themselves lacking confidence in administrative and leadership skills and being unaware of the many associated responsibilities. They may be faced with quality improvement issues (eg, seclusion and restraint reduction, programming, and staff morale or other challenges). This article provides an overview of leadership and administrative responsibilities associated with medical directorship on inpatient child and adolescent psychiatric services. Issues and challenges unique to academic settings and the private sector are examined (government-funded leadership roles in child and adolescent psychiatry are described elsewhere in this issue). Following this is an introduction to approaching projects related to organizational change and quality improvement.

[a] Child and Adolescent Inpatient Services, Department of Psychiatry, CB # 7160, University of North Carolina, Chapel Hill, NC 27599–7160, USA
[b] Rush University Medical Center, 120 East Ogden Avenue, Suite 222, Hinsdale, IL 60521, USA
[c] Division of Child and Adolescent Psychiatry, Cincinnati Children's Hospital Medical Center, University of Cincinnati, 3333 Burnet Avenue, ML 3014, Cincinnati, OH 45229, USA
[d] Maryville Academy, 555 Wilson Lane, Des Plaines, IL 60016, USA
* Corresponding author.
E-mail address: Erin_malloy@med.unc.edu (E. Malloy).

Child Adolesc Psychiatric Clin N Am 19 (2010) 1–19
doi:10.1016/j.chc.2009.08.008
1056-4993/09/$ – see front matter © 2010 Elsevier Inc. All rights reserved.

childpsych.theclinics.com

THE ACADEMIC ACUTE INPATIENT CHILD AND ADOLESCENT PSYCHIATRIST

Although many of the issues faced in child and adolescent psychiatric inpatient leadership positions in the private sector are shared in the academic setting, there are several aspects that are unique. The transition from resident to attending or even medical director in the same program has its challenges; transitioning to a new institution has its own issues. Mastery of clinical expertise and the aforementioned administrative and leadership skills is demanding in its own right. In some academic institutions, the administrative role is diluted to some extent by distinct, parallel leadership among nursing staff, social workers, and ancillary services. Establishing working relationships and skills in team building is imperative. Another distinctive feature of the inpatient medical director in the academic setting is the additional missions of teaching and research. Furthermore, career development and academic promotion are key but often underemphasized concerns for the academic inpatient child and adolescent psychiatrist. The discussion also presents strategies to deal with difficulties in these areas and to prevent and manage burnout.

The Transition from Resident to Attending Psychiatrist: Potential Challenges

Psychiatry residents are often recruited by their training programs to take on faculty positions. The plight of the junior faculty member in the challenging role of the psychiatric inpatient unit director was introduced over 20 years ago by Leibenluft and colleagues,[2] including the observation of high turnover rates of junior faculty in these positions. Indeed, with continued work in an academic department come additional duties in terms of hospital committees, medical school and residency training responsibilities, and the like. In addition, faculty may be promoted to positions that leave them with little time for their intensive clinical duties. Many child psychiatry residents have spent several months working in the acute inpatient setting during their training and have developed confidence in their clinical skills in this arena. The transition into a clinical leadership position from training may have some pitfalls. For example, the relationships the physician has with staff may need to become more professional. Staff may need to adjust to the physician's new, more authoritative role. The physician may be dismayed by not being taken as seriously as they would like to be. The physician may have difficulty being assertive in these situations. Addressing this particular concern early on is important; ideally, preparing for the new role with conversations with staff and staff leadership before the changeover, modeling leadership, and team-building skills in the process.

A somewhat different problem is faced by the resident taking on an inpatient leadership role at a different institution. In this case, staff's lack of familiarity with the physician may lead to lack of confidence in the physician's clinical and leadership skills. In this case, a designated orientation period where the physician can learn the procedures and policies of the hospital, get a feel for staff concerns, program strengths, and areas in need of improvement, is advisable. Spending some time in "data collection mode" before an actual start date may prove to be quite useful. In both of these situations (and for any transition into a new inpatient leadership position) negotiating for a transition period without clinical responsibilities is recommended. Most inpatient medical directors wish to portray themselves as being approachable to their staff. Although this is important, it can become a proverbial "slippery-slope" where the physician-leader becomes so available that work responsibilities infringe on personal time in an unhealthy manner. Balancing approachability with establishing boundaries is a challenge, but a very important one. This is discussed in more detail in the section related to managing stress and preventing burn-out.

A new medical director, with admirable standards for excellence, may also become susceptible to taking on additional clinical responsibilities that may belong to other members of the treatment team. In the academic setting, this risk is compounded by the recent and familiar role as a resident physician; here the attending may take on more of what should be the resident's responsibilities. Being helpful and role-modeling for residents is important. The resident in such a situation, however, may miss out on opportunities for active learning and developing their own clinical skills.[1] It may be useful for the attending to reflect on how their own role models and mentors handled this balance and how prepared they felt as residents to manage clinical situations based on the attending supervision they obtained in their training. Such self-evaluation may also reveal underlying insecurities or anxieties regarding competency in the physician leader role. Increased self-awareness is a major step in managing stress related to this work.

Defining the Leadership Role

The complex organization of leadership in academic institutions presents further concerns for the child and adolescent inpatient psychiatrist. It is important to determine the sources of one's salary: some inpatient academic child and adolescent psychiatrists are paid by the hospital, some by the medical school, some by state funds, or any combination thereof. Academic hospitals may differ significantly in their leadership structure (eg, parallel leadership structures among physicians, nursing, social work, and ancillary services may dilute the medical director's authority to lead the team). In such cases it is imperative for the physician to demonstrate assertiveness in making treatment decisions and skills in team-building so as to gain the respect of other team members. It may be useful for the physician in such a situation to cultivate their role as a leader before taking on major initiatives for change. As one resource, Kotter's[3,4] work on leading change is quite informative in the development of leadership teams, understanding dynamics, and in planning and effecting change. It should be emphasized that in any case, regardless of direct leadership structure, responsibility for outcomes ultimately may rest on the physician, underscoring the importance of the development of a leadership persona.

Career Development: A Triple (or Quadruple) Threat?

Development of clinical expertise and administrative and leadership skills are very important tasks for the early career child and adolescent psychiatrist. In the academic setting, the additional roles of educator and researcher may be difficult to balance. The charge of delegating clinical responsibilities to residents in the provision of training is an important one in the development of the faculty member's role as teacher. With full understanding of the time constraints involved, the academic inpatient child psychiatrist would do well to identify opportunities to teach in the context of the provision of clinical care and leadership. Modeling and observing interviewing skills is one salient example of this, given recent developments in requirements for board certification in child and adolescent psychiatry, which include several observed interviews during training for residents to become board eligible.[5] Determining the educational needs of child psychiatry residents, general psychiatry residents at various levels, and medical students is imperative. For example, the educational goals in the interview of an adolescent may include establishing rapport and asking about substance abuse and sexuality for the medical student; the psychiatric interview and presentation skills for the general resident; and developing a formulation, differential diagnosis, and treatment plan for the child psychiatry resident. Case conferences that enable trainees and treatment team members to discuss findings, diagnoses, and treatment planning may also be useful in both a clinical and educational sense. The thoughtful assignment of clinical questions for research and the discussion of findings from literature searches may be used in this manner.

Participation in research and scholarly activities may seem difficult for the academic inpatient child psychiatrist. Again, the pairing of these endeavors with clinical duties can be practical and worthwhile. The creation of teaching or orientation documents may be used as documentation of scholarly activity for the busy clinician with little time to pursue publication. With that in mind, such documents should be crafted well and with clear identification of references, authorship, and creation date. Furthermore, many academic inpatient child and adolescent psychiatrists are asked to give lectures to students, residents, and colleagues; lecture documents may also be edited for this purpose. As far as clinical research related to inpatient work is concerned, Brown[6] describes creating an inpatient database as a means of obtaining prospective data to address research questions in a clinically and professionally meaningful way. Chart reviews and questionnaires of patients, families, or staff are other means of pursuing research. One may also pursue educational research by creating surveys for students and trainees.

It is not surprising that, with the multiple demands described previously, the level of intensity of the cases encountered, and the steep learning curves in numerous areas, the early career child psychiatrist choosing an academic inpatient leadership role is susceptible to stress and a phenomenon known as "burnout." Burnout can lead to the unfortunate consequence of a truncated academic career. Brown,[6] in his article on the inpatient database, also addresses the issue of "burnout" for psychiatrists who do inpatient work in academic settings. Development of mentoring relationships has been shown to enhance productivity in academic medicine, not only in research publications,[7] but in retention of faculty and cost-effectiveness through a formal mentoring program as described by Wingard and colleagues.[8] Mentoring may also enhance quality of life for academic physicians. Zerzan and colleagues[9] offer guidance to junior faculty perusing mentorship relationships, encouraging the junior faculty member to take a proactive role in "managing up" in the mentoring relationship. Moss and colleagues[10] describe a peer mentoring approach more specific to academic psychiatrists with quite favorable responses from its participants. Some departments have formal mentoring programs. Regardless, it is recommended that academic inpatient child and adolescent psychiatrists develop some constructive and supportive relationships with colleagues to assist with career development; provide guidance in clinical, administrative, and research issues; and prevent burnout.

Although certainly the academic setting poses challenges, opportunities to learn, teach, and discover abound. The private sector offers some benefits, such as increased salary and independence. There are many distinct aspects of clinical leadership in the private psychiatric hospital setting that warrant discussion. A case illustration is presented to highlight important issues.

THE INPATIENT CHILD PSYCHIATRIST IN THE PRIVATE SECTOR
Case Illustration

Dr Davis is a child and adolescent psychiatrist who had recently joined a freestanding private psychiatric hospital as its medical director. She had recently completed her child psychiatry residency training and had been working as a junior attending on an inpatient unit of a large university hospital. The private hospital opportunity presented her with a significant increase in compensation and growth potential. During her contract negotiations, she was informed that this was a full-time, salaried position and her responsibilities would include a caseload of 12 patients in addition to her administrative duties. She was told that the hospital administration wanted to move toward employing physicians, which was a shift from its previous model, which had been along the lines of having independent contractual relationships with physicians.

The hospital was a privately owned, 120-bed acute inpatient facility and had recently been purchased by a corporation that owned several other hospitals in the state. Dr Davis was faced with her first challenge 2 months after her start in the form of a Joint Commission survey. Her previous experiences with such surveys had left her with the impression that physicians had minimal involvement in the survey process and that it was handled primarily by nursing leadership and administration. She was surprised to see, however, that the hospital administration and the surveyors expected her full participation. She sat in on the introductory and exit interviews and spent an entire day with the physician surveyor. She felt unprepared for this process and had to defer many questions to her medical staff coordinator. For example, during a review of the credentialing process she was asked about the mechanisms used to ensure that physicians practice within their scope of privileges. Another area of uncertainty for Dr Davis arose when one of the surveyors had commented that the current model of paying clinical directors stipends could be interpreted as a "kickback" for patient referrals. An additional topic that was discussed involved the role of medical leadership in organization performance improvement activities to improve quality of care. The surveyor made a comment that there was little evidence that the organized medical staff was actively providing leadership in "measuring, assessing and improving processes that would result in an improved quality of care and treatment."

A few months later, Dr Davis was faced with another crisis: an incident involving two adolescents engaging in sexual activity on the adolescent unit of the hospital. Two days later, the Department of Public Health made an unannounced visit to the hospital to perform a "focused review" as a result of the incident. Again, Dr Davis had never gone through a process like this and was asked about her role and that of the organized medical leadership in response to a critical or sentinel event. Specifically, they wanted to know if the physician leadership was involved in the root cause analysis of the event.

Dr Davis was finding it increasingly challenging to manage her clinical duties because of her administrative load. As the medical director, she served as chair for most of the medical staff committees. She had never chaired committees before and found it difficult to make these meetings productive. Dr Davis had numerous discussions with the hospital administration about her concerns about many of the issues she had come across during her employment. She eventually decided to resign from the hospital because of a lack of agreement between her and the administration.

This case highlights some important issues and challenges faced by psychiatrists entering into leadership positions at private for-profit psychiatric hospitals:

1. Lack of adequate administrative and leadership training during residency and fellowship.[1]
2. Potential conflict of interest when working for a for-profit hospital that has an obligation to its investors. Under these circumstances a physician might be placed in a situation where there is pressure from the administration to increase profits at the cost of quality of care.
3. Ensuring adequate time to perform the administrative duties without compromising clinical care of patients. It is important when negotiating a contract to allocate sufficient time toward administrative duties.
4. Familiarity with health care laws.

There has been an increase in the number of private psychiatric hospitals and corporations involved in acute inpatient psychiatry. Many of these hospitals have child and adolescent units. It is important for child and adolescent psychiatrists considering or entering into medical director positions in the private psychiatric acute inpatient setting to familiarize themselves with some basics. An understanding of the financial arrangements of the hospital with physicians and referral agencies is critical. In addition, it is important to study the organizational chart of the hospital.

Organizational Structure of the Private, For-profit Psychiatric Hospital

Although numerous organizational models exist,[11] many private psychiatric hospitals have an organizational structure that can be divided into three areas: (1) the governing body, (2) medical staff, and (3) administration and leadership.

Governing body

The governing body (or board) is ultimately responsible and accountable for the quality and effectiveness of patient care services provided throughout the facility. In addition, it is responsible for ensuring that a uniform balance of patient care is provided to all patients. The governing board typically delegates responsibility for the development and implementation of the facility's performance improvement plan to administration and the medical staff. Delegation of authority is established in accordance with medical staff bylaws and rules and regulations and hospital policies and procedures. The governing board regularly reviews reports of performance improvement activities to assess the effectiveness of the program in meeting its goals.

Medical staff

The organized medical staff takes a leadership role in performance improvement activities to improve quality of care, treatment and services, and patient safety. It provides leadership for measuring, assessing, and improving processes that primarily depend on the activities of one or more licensed independent practitioners and other practitioners credentialed and privileged through the medical staff process. These processes often include medical assessment and treatment of patients, use of medication, appropriateness of clinical practice patterns, and significant departures from established patterns of clinical practice.

Additionally, the organized medical staff may also participate in the improvement of other patient care processes, such as education of patients and families; coordination of patient care with other practitioners and hospital personnel; and accurate, timely, and legible completion of patients' medical records.

The medical staff is commonly led by a medical executive committee, which is responsible for the ongoing measurement, assessment, and improvement of activities provided by the medical staff, and those activities provided by nursing, support staff, and contracted services. The medical executive committee performs the following types of activities:

- Review and response to reports from medical staff committees and other departments or services
- Determination of ongoing evaluation of a practitioner's competence when findings are relevant to the quality of professional services provided by individuals with clinical privileges
- Communication of findings, conclusions, recommendations, and actions taken to improve facility performance to the appropriate committee, program, or service and to appropriate staff members, medical staff members, and the governing body.

Administration and leadership

Administration, or leadership, is accountable for planning, directing, integrating, and improving patient care services provided throughout the facility. Leaders may include the chief executive officer, chief operating officer, medical director, and chief nursing officer, or combinations thereof.[11] It is the responsibility of leadership to become educated in the approaches and methods of performance improvement. It is this education and the assimilation of the principles of quality leadership and performance improvement that support process improvement activities throughout the facility. Leadership is responsible for the implementation of the performance improvement plan and ongoing performance improvement activities through the performance improvement committee. Examples of processes of leadership that are typically used include.

Planning and designing services: Provide a collaborative process for developing long-range, strategic, and operational plans; service design; resource allocation; and facility policies.

Directing services: Ensure that patient care and support services are well organized and staffed in a manner commensurate with the scope of services offered by each program.

Integrating and coordinating services: Communicate objectives and coordinate efforts to integrate patient care and support services throughout the facility.

Improving performance: Establish expectations, plans, and priorities for facility-wide programs and services. Ensure implementation of processes to design, measure, analyze, improve, and maintain the performance of the facility's governance, management, clinical, and support processes.

Role of the Medical Director

The role of the medical director as an executive leader must be distinguished from management and staff activities. This is necessary to enable the physician leader to move away from a "crisis response" mode and to establish long-term goals. The first step is a detailed job description that delineates the role of the medical director in leading medical staff affairs. The medical director should, through this step, become a part of the senior leadership of the organization and be a contributor to the strategic direction of the organization.

The physician leader also must ensure a meaningful and consistent engagement of medical staff in performance improvement activities. This can be achieved by having physicians serve in leadership roles in organizational activities around infection control, health information management, patient safety, and quality management. They provide leadership for measuring, assessing, and improving processes that include medical assessment and treatment of patients, use of medication, appropriateness of clinical practice patterns, and significant departures from established patterns of clinical practice.

Involvement of the medical director with regulatory and accreditation bodies

There has been an increase in scrutiny and regulation of free-standing psychiatric hospitals. The standards applicable to medical surgical facilities are not always helpful in determining the quality of care at a psychiatric facility. The Joint Commission and the National Association of Psychiatric Health Systems, the National Association of State Mental Health Program Directors, and the National Association of State Mental Health Program Directors Research Institute have finished work on a set of core performance measures for hospital-based inpatient psychiatric services, which has been piloted. Work on specifications for the following measures has been completed[12]:

- Admission screening for violence risk, substance use, psychologic trauma history, and patient strengths completed
- Hours of physical restraint use
- Hours of seclusion use
- Patients discharged on multiple antipsychotic medications
- Patients discharged on multiple antipsychotic medications with appropriate justification
- Postdischarge continuing care plan created
- Postdischarge continuing care plan transmitted to next level of care provider on discharge

A number of these organizations provide accessible and useful information for the physician leader in the child and adolescent psychiatric inpatient setting. Such resources include the US Department of Health and Human Services—the Office of the Inspector General[13] and Centers for Medicare and Medicaid Services,[14] the Joint Commission,[15] and the National Association of Psychiatric Health Systems.[16] In addition, the American Academy of Child and Adolescent Psychiatry is in the process of reviewing clinical guidelines and practice parameters related to the psychiatric inpatient care of children and adolescents (unpublished data).

Involvement with managed care entities and Medicaid reimbursement may be yet another responsibility of the medical director in the child-adolescent psychiatric inpatient setting. Negotiation and understanding of contracts between the hospital and insurance companies and a thorough understanding of Medicaid reimbursement[17] are recommended.

Health Care Laws

The medical director of a private psychiatric hospital needs to be familiar with certain health care laws, including Stark law, antikickback statutes, and the Emergency Medical Treatment and Active Labor Act.

Stark law

Generally speaking, the Stark law, which can be found in Section 1877 of the Social Security Act,[18] prohibits a physician from referring Medicare or Medicaid program patients for certain "designated health services" to an entity with which the physician or an immediate family member has a "financial relationship." The "designated health services" covered by the Stark law include inpatient hospital services and hence apply to acute inpatient psychiatric treatment of children and adolescents. Any physicians who are investors in hospitals or who have other financial incentives should be aware of any potential conflicts. This law has undergone numerous revisions; it is important for the physician leader in the private setting to remain abreast.[19]

Federal antikickback law

The federal antikickback statute prohibits individuals or entities to pay, offer to pay, solicit, or accept any type of remuneration, direct or indirect, in exchange for the referral of or recommending or arranging for referral of patients, items, or services reimbursed by a health care program. Some courts have interpreted the law to cover any arrangement in which one purpose of the remuneration is to induce or compensate for referrals. Continual review of such legislation is important.[19]

Emergency medical treatment and active labor act

The Emergency Medical Treatment and Active Labor Act is a statute that governs when and how a patient may be refused treatment or transferred from one hospital to another when he or she is in an unstable medical condition.[20] The Emergency Medical Treatment and Active Labor Act was passed as part of the Consolidated Omnibus Budget Reconciliation Act of 1986, and it is sometimes referred to as "the COBRA law." Any patient who "comes to the emergency department" requesting "examination or treatment for a medical condition" must be provided with "an appropriate medical screening examination" to determine if he or she is suffering from an "emergency medical condition." If they are, then the hospital is obligated to either provide them with treatment until they are stable or to transfer them to another hospital in conformance with the statute's directives. A medical director of a free-standing psychiatric hospital must ensure that patients who "walk into" the hospital in unstable conditions are assessed by qualified professionals and provided the appropriate level of care.[21]

Comprehensive understanding of the multifaceted role of the private sector inpatient child psychiatrist is imperative to success in this arena. Preparation and study of such career opportunities in the private setting should prevent unfortunate outcomes, such as that of Dr Davis in the case illustration.

Although roles of the inpatient child psychiatrist in the academic and private sectors possess some differing characteristics, common themes regarding the development of leadership skills, managing change,[3,4] and continuing quality improvement in services remain. The final section of this article focuses on quality improvement in the acute inpatient child psychiatric setting.

QUALITY IMPROVEMENT AND LEADERSHIP ON THE CHILD INPATIENT PSYCHIATRIC UNIT

Leadership on the inpatient psychiatric unit has many challenges because unit directors and physician leaders not only need to be abreast of the most advanced clinical techniques to treat patient illness, but also be adept with management techniques to oversee a complex system providing care to acute severely ill patients. Typical training of physicians offers little experience in leadership methods. Emphasis in medical training and research has been to explore disorder-specific pathology, improve clinical recognition, and enhance treatment techniques to improve the quality of care. Psychiatry research often focuses on new pharmacotherapy interventions, enhanced psychotherapy techniques, or improvement to existing therapies, all of which have led to significant and at times dramatic improvements in patient care outcomes. Perhaps underrecognized have been the opportunities to improve the quality of care that exists outside the provision of new specific psychotherapies or advanced pharmacotherapy.[22] Focusing on such issues as improving care processes, reduction in variation, coordination of care teams, and systems approach to care have led to great improvements in many areas of medicine. These improvements frequently stem from highly reliable consistent performance of current care techniques and current technology. Recent examples include dramatic reductions in pediatric ventilator-associated pneumonia and rates of central line infections.[23,24]

Mental health care has lagged behind other fields in medicine in embracing and incorporating quality improvement initiatives into daily care processes.[25] To provide psychiatric services to an often complicated population, the inpatient psychiatric unit spans a complex array of activities, systems, personnel, disciplines, and processes that all have the potential to be evaluated, revised, and improved to enhance the quality of care for patients. Leadership of the inpatient psychiatric unit goes beyond a working knowledge of best practices and treatment of specific conditions, and requires an understanding of a broader systematic framework in which clinical care is delivered. Approaching the role of leadership through adaption of principles of structured quality improvement provides the means to the leader and frontline provider to improve quality, enhance patient outcomes, increase satisfaction, reduce variation, and diminish waste.[26,27]

Quality management science in general industry has served as the model for improvement science in medicine.[28] The underlying principles of the models, based on the work of early industry quality experts, such as Juran[29] and Deming,[30] include techniques from psychology, engineering, statistics, and systems theory. In existence for over 60 years, these methods undergo persistent revision and improvement. Resulting successes in productivity, satisfaction, and quality has led to widespread adoption and implementation of quality improvement techniques and principles by industry.

The Institute of Medicine[31] pointed out that despite the ability of the United States to provide outstanding health care, there is a tremendous gap in what patients actually do receive versus what they could or should receive. As indicated in this report, these gaps and failures were found in all types of services, including those of behavioral health. More recently, organized psychiatry has called to apply the Institute of Medicine framework of improving health care to mental health and substance abuse treatment.[32,33] Serving as director of specific system of care, such as an inpatient psychiatric unit, puts the leader in a position of attempting to bridge these gaps and ensure that patients receive the care they should get on a consistent high-quality basis. The following discussion identifies a few of the specific areas of science and quality improvement that leaders may use to enhance the provision of care on inpatient psychiatric services.

Project Models and Problem-solving

Leadership of the inpatient psychiatric unit is persistently confronted by solving problems in the clinical process. Common difficulties include variations of care by providers; occurrence of adverse safety events; underuse, overuse, and misuse of specific interventions; and general errors in care. Frequently, the initial response to problems is to identify individuals at fault and have specific corrective action. Work by Juran[29] and others point out that processes are much more frequently at fault. The potential to diminish mistakes and eliminate errors actually involves improving the systems through which the work is done, not in changing employees. For example, a physician struggles with appropriate admission orders when there has not been an appropriate hand-off in care or a psychiatric nurse is unable to provide appropriate psychotherapeutic response to a crisis when treatment planning is inadequate. Leaders must recognize that most problems in medical care are caused by the systems in which individuals operate.[34] Laying cause at the feet of specific individuals does not typically lead to improvement. This is only gained by focus on the system.

Inpatient Leadership and Clinical Microsystems

Assuming leadership of an inpatient unit puts one in charge of a clinical microsystem. The clinical microsystem is where patients, families, and health care teams meet. More specifically, as described by Nelson and coworkers,[35] the clinical microsystem is a small group of people who work together on a regular basis to provide care to specific populations of patients. It has clinical and business aims, linked processes, a shared information environment, and produces services and care. Microsystems evolve over time and often are embedded in larger organizations. They are complex systems, and as such they must do primary work associated with core aims, meet the needs of internal staff, and maintain themselves over time as clinical units.[35] Essentially, microsystems form the basic structure of health care delivery in hospital settings. The concept for microsystems in health care originated from the work in the corporate world of Quinn.[36] His work in examining high-functioning organizations was aimed at finding the common themes that led to their success. These leading organizations have a continued focus on the front line interface relationship between the organization service and the needs of individual customers. He identified these as the minimum replicable unit embedded in the service process. Child and adolescent inpatient clinical microsystems are composed of the identified child adolescent patient, their families or guardians, physicians, nurses, nurses aids, mental health specialists, unit administrators, social workers, care managers, and support personnel. At the microsystem level, patients and families present with various needs, and processes begin to assess these needs, diagnose underlying conditions, formulate problem lists, develop treatment plans, provide treatment, and determine disposition. There are handoffs to follow-up care and education of patients and families. Supporting the microsystem are multiple processes, such as pharmacy, patient finance and billing, scheduling, and medical records. From these interactions are produced patient clinical outcomes and satisfaction, staff satisfaction and development, and status of the unit in regards to reputation and finances.[35] It is the point of where systems of health care and patient needs come together that determines such issues as safety and quality.[37] It is also the area where most workplace motivators and demotivators are found, leading to determination of the provider's success and satisfaction. Leadership must understand that the system is an interdependent group of people and processes working together toward a common purpose. Understanding this system and developing a plan to improve the system is the key responsibility of leadership.[38,39] Leadership must integrate diverse components so they serve not only the microsystem, but the whole organization. It is not the performance of individual components but the success of the organization, and specifically the microsystem, that determines the quality of service and potential outcomes. The quality of service delivered depends of the successful integration of diverse components, processes, and personnel.

Leadership should embrace specific qualities to enhance the functional status of the microsystem. The overall areas of focus are illustrated by a detailed description of characteristics of successful microsystems by a series of articles by the Joint Commission.[35,37–44] These characteristics include leadership that demonstrates a constancy of purpose with establishment of clear goals that fosters a positive culture and advocates for the microsystem in the larger organization. Leadership must foster the development of a culture where diverse staff has shared beliefs and values and all clinical mission contributions are respected and seen as an important component to success of the microsystem. Leadership advocates for organizational support and provision of resources for the microsystem to accomplish their goals. The system of care is patient focused and patient care is the primary concern and purpose. Successful microsystems include a staff focus and culture that highly regards performance, professional growth, and continuing education. These systems recognize that there is a high interdependence of the care team with a multidisciplinary approach, respect for each other, and a willingness to help. These highly successful systems also have appropriate information technology and information processes that provide feedback regarding performance and process improvement to the microsystem so it may adapt, develop, and improve.

Leading Improvement

Work of leadership on inpatient units includes facing the challenge of ongoing and newly presenting problems, continuous improvement of care processes, enhancing the resources to support the work on the unit, and diminishing waste with the goal of improving outcomes for patients. Identification of a group of people representing the multidisciplinary nature of the care teams and assembling them into an improvement team is an initial step in enhancing quality. Typical teams are based on the work by Juran[29] and others[28,45] and are composed of three to nine people who are involved in the daily care processes. Team members represent the multiple disciplines involved in care and bring forth the ideas from each of these disciplines to be discussed and explored in the team process. Teams require cooperation that extends beyond typical boundaries because many interdependent resources and skills are required to provide and improve health care.

Development of the purpose of the team and aim for the improvement process is critical. To be most effective, one must be specific, have measurable data, be actionable such that the microsystem or care providers can impact the problem, be relevant to improving the processes or outcomes under investigation, and be time limited.[45]

Case Illustration Part 1

An adolescent inpatient psychiatric unit has created a continuous process to try to decrease the amount of aggressive episodes by patients, the number of physical interventions by staff, and the frequency of staff injury. Initial improvement work had developed an instrument examining specific elements in the psychiatric history that identified at the time of admission 90% of the adolescents who had subsequent aggressive episodes on the inpatient unit that required seclusion, mechanical restraint, or physical hold. Typically, these patients had extensive past histories of aggressive behavior, and high levels of past and observed impulsivity. Several initiatives to address the problem were underway with one element focusing on medication administration. Inpatient nursing staff reported to the physicians that there was extreme variation in the practice of PRN medication for severe aggressive behavior on the inpatient units, especially in patients with bipolar spectrum illness and psychosis. Also noted was extreme variation of when or if nurses offer an appropriate PRN medication when a patient is escalating. The clinical team wanted to standardize the practice throughout the multidisciplinary physician group that admitted to this unit and have consistent triggers by staff on when to offer a PRN medication. The overall goal of this group was to decrease the aggressive episodes requiring physical interventions by adapting a standardized approach to the type of medication offered and when it was offered. The emphasis for the group was to offer the "right" medicine at the "right" time to prevent escalation to severe aggression. The specific aim was to decrease by 25% the occurrence of aggressive episodes requiring physical intervention because of development and implementation of appropriate PRN medication program for aggression in high-risk patients in 6 months. This aim was time-limited and thought to have actionable items and directly pertinent to the overall goal of the care group. After establishment of the purpose of the team, overall goal, and specific aim for intervention and evaluation the team must fully describe the process, determine measurements, and engage in cycles of improvement.

Describing the Process

After description of goals and scope of project, a graphic representation of the processes involved is needed. Flow charts graphically represent the series of events or steps in the work process. An additional level of description is a failure mode analysis, which involves examination of processes to identify needed improvements that are thought to reduce the chance of unintended adverse events or failure of the process (**Fig. 1**).[46] This method incorporates delineating steps of a current or proposed clinical process and evaluating what events or situations at each step may cause failure. These failures may be human errors, equipment problems, communication difficulties, missing or misplaced supplies, or any other obstacles that might disrupt the process. The severity of each failure mode is typically ranked in its' severity and potential frequency, resulting in design interventions to avoid potential failures. The goal of failure mode analysis is based on the concepts developed by the aerospace industry and involves identifying potential mistakes or obstacles that will happen before they do happen and determining whether the consequences of these mistakes are tolerable or intolerable.[46,47] The reliability of successful completion of a multistep process requires that the performance of each step have an extremely high reliability. The flow chart with examination of potential failure is used to address the issue of reliability. In a six-step process where each step has a 90% chance of successful completion, the reliability of all steps being accomplished hovers at 50%. Designing a high-reliability process requires close attention to each step to ensure its' successful completion.

Case Illustration Part 2

The unit treatment team mapped major process steps, potential failures, and interventions for the new process of identifying high aggression risk patients and institution of standardized PRN protocol. Each step in the process needed to achieve high reliability for success of the overall program. The improvement teams used multiple small tests of change for each process step.

Improvement Model

Models for improvement in health care have been adapted from the corporate world and industrial quality management described by early leaders, such as Deming[30] and Shewhart.[48] These models have been adapted for health care and detailed by Langley and coworkers.[49] The model begins with several questions that need to be answered: what is one trying to accomplish, how will one know that a change is an improvement, and what changes can one make that will result in improvement. This leads to the "Plan, Do, Study, Act" (PDSA) cycle of improvement (**Fig. 2**). Using the cycle, planned changes are made in the current system, effects are measured, and determination is made if the process is moving closer to the stated aim. The results from alterations in the process are examined and this information is used to engage in another rapid cycle change. Typical cycles are small scale, rapid, and incremental. An example of a small test of change is demonstrated in **Box 1**. A typical improvement project may have several PDSA cycles in operations, each exploring different elements or steps of the overall process that is being optimized. Having direct front-line care staff involved in or leading the PDSA model often gives most valuable information. Leadership on the unit must continually refocus improvement teams and the clinical microsystem to engage in the use of PDSA improvement cycles, posting current changes and engaging people in the process, obtaining their feedback, learning from their experiences, assisting with future cycles, and enhancing the chance to lead to the gradual improvement desired.

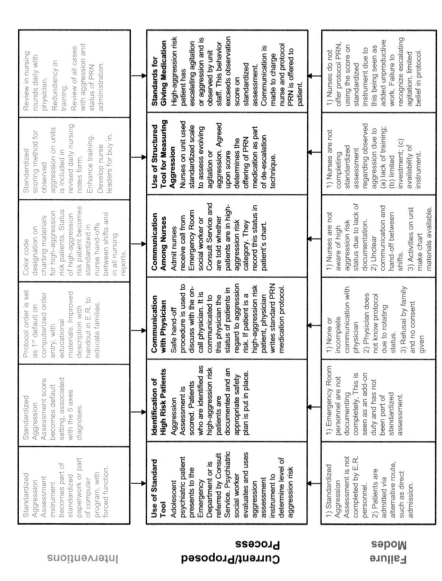

Fig. 1. Flow chart of care process with observed, anticipated failures, and proposed interventions to avoid failure.

Sample Model of Improvement

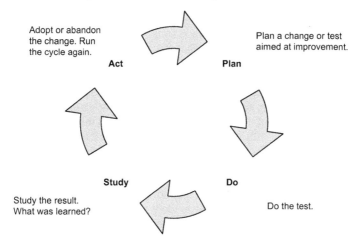

Adopt or abandon the change. Run the cycle again.

Act

Plan a change or test aimed at improvement.

Plan

Study

Study the result. What was learned?

Do

Do the test.

Questions to Determine Directives of Improvement

1. What are we trying to accomplish?
2. How will we know that a change is an improvement?
3. What changes can we make that will result in improvement?

Fig. 2. Sample model of improvement. Shewhart WA, Deming WE. The improvement guide: a practical approach to enhancing organizational performance. In: Langley GJ, Nolan KM, Nolan TW, et al. Healthcare. 1996. p. 49. (*Adapted from* Langley GJ, Nolan KM, Nolan W, et al. The Improvement Guide. San Francisco, CA: Jossey-Bass, 1996.)

Box 1
Hypothetical example of PDSA test of change report

Small test of change report, test cycle 1: start date = 7/1/07 and end date = 7/15/07.

Specific aim: To decrease by 25% the occurrence of aggressive episodes requiring physical intervention caused by the development and implementation of appropriate PRN medication for aggression in high-risk patients over a period of 6 months.

Objective of this test of change: To properly identify high aggressive risk patients as standard procedure at intake assessment.

Plan and prediction: By revising the intake form in electronic medical record to include aggression assessment and having drop-down scoring boxes directly following DSM-IV axes diagnoses, compliance will improve to 90%.

Do: Evaluate all intake forms to inpatient psychiatry over a 2-week period. Determine number of charts with properly indicated aggression risk.

Study: Appropriate completion of assessment occurred with 80% compliance on weekdays and less than 30% on weekends.

Act: Investigation of why this is not used more appropriately on weekends and identify specific individuals not in compliance during week days. Educate PRN and weekend staff in use of protocol. Future PDSA investigation of forced function on electronic documentation to improve compliance.

Case Illustration Part 3

PDSA cycles regarding identification of patients may be underway while improvements in clinical handoffs are also being studied and revised using the same process. Multiple PDSA cycles where used for each step of the new care process until the reliability of each step approached 100%. Simultaneously, there was ongoing monitoring of aggressive episodes requiring seclusion, restraint, or physical hold. Episodes and rates were posted quarterly on all units in the form of run charts to monitor progress of the overall program. Reduction of aggressive episodes approached 40%.

A child psychiatrist acting in a leadership position for the inpatient service is responsible for the development of the unit and its' contribution to the overlying organization. Organizations successful with improvement efforts, as described by Plsek,[28] have four key habits: (1) the habit of viewing clinical practice as a process that incorporates the need for complex coordination of people and systems; (2) the habit for evidence-based medicine to diminish the variation in health care and drive care processes to be those that are most effective; (3) the habit of collaborative learning where building and knowledge of systems, and interdependent processes are not found in scientific literature, but in the skills and knowledge of the participants in the system; and (4) the habit for change where leaders provide a culture and support that encourages and requires ongoing change to gain new knowledge and improve performance.[28]

SUMMARY

Child psychiatrists who pursue leadership roles in acute inpatient settings may find the opportunities to hone skills in leadership, administration, and clinical expertise. With a full appreciation of needs for support and mentoring, organizational structure, applicable health care legislation, the accreditation process, and economic issues physician leaders in these roles can be very well prepared to make appropriate career choices and improve their job satisfaction. Understanding issues related to organizational change and quality improvement processes can result in improved quality of care, better outcomes for patients, and a sense of competency in one's leadership abilities. Combining the clinical and leadership responsibilities with an academic career can be possible given proper planning and application of educational and research endeavors to the clinical and administrative work. Completing this necessary groundwork is critical for the physician leader on the child-adolescent psychiatric inpatient unit to achieve career fulfillment.

REFERENCES

1. Stubbe D. Preparation for practice: child and adolescent psychiatry graduates' assessment of training experiences. J Am Acad Child Adolesc Psychiatry 2002;41(2):131–9.
2. Leibenluft E, Summergrad P, Tasman A. The academic dilemma of the inpatient unit director. Am J Psychiatry 1989;146:73–6.
3. Kotter JP. Leading change. Harv Bus Rev 2007;85(1):96–103.
4. Kotter J, Rathgeber H. Our iceberg is melting. New York: St. Martin's Press; 2005.
5. American Board of Psychiatry and Neurology. Clinical skills evaluation of residents in child and adolescent psychiatry. 2009. Available at: http://www.abpn.com/downloads/forms/CAP_CSV_Instructional_Guide.pdf. Accessed April 13, 2009.
6. Brown GR. The inpatient database as a technique to prevent junior faculty burnout. Acad Psychiatry 1990;14:224–9.

7. Steiner JF, Curtis P, Lamphear BP, et al. Assessing the role of influential mentors in the research development of primary care fellows. Acad Med 2004;79(9):865–72.
8. Wingard DL, Garman KA, Reznik V. Facilitating faculty success: outcomes and cost benefit of the UCSD National Center of Leadership in Academic Medicine. Acad Med 2004;79(Suppl 10):S9–11.
9. Zerzan JT, Hess R, Schur E, et al. Making the most of mentors: a guide for mentees. Acad Med 2009;84(1):140–4.
10. Moss J, Teshima J, Leszcz M. Peer group mentoring of junior faculty. Acad Psychiatry 2008;32(3):230–5.
11. Sharfstein S, Schwartz H. Administration and leadership. In: Sharfstein SS, Dickerson FB, Oldham JM, editors. Textbook of hospital psychiatry. Arlington (VA): American Psychiatric Publishing, Inc; 2009. p. 357–69.
12. The Joint Commission. National hospital inpatient quality measures- hospital based inpatient psychiatric services (HBIPS) core measure set. Available at: http://www.jointcommission.org/PerformanceMeasurement/PerformanceMeasurement/Hospital+Based+Inpatient+Psychiatric+Services.htm. Last Updated 3/6/09. Accessed April 14, 2009.
13. US Department of Health and Human Services. Office of Inspector General. Available at: http://www.oig.hhs.gov. Accessed April 14, 2009.
14. US Department of Health and Human Services. Centers for Medicare and Medicaid Services. Available at: http://www.cms.hhs.gov/. Accessed April 14, 2009.
15. Joint Commission. Comprehensive accreditation manual for behavioral health care (CAMBHC). Available at: http://www.jcrinc.com/Joint-Commission-Requirements/Behavioral-Health-Care. Last updated June 13, 2009. Accessed July 27, 2009.
16. National Association of Psychiatric Health Systems. Available at: http://www.naphs.org/quality/HBIPS.html. Accessed April 14, 2009.
17. US Department of Health and Human Services, Centers for Medicare and Medicaid Services. Available at: http://www.cms.hhs.gov/home/medicaid.asp. Accessed April 14, 2009.
18. US Social Security Administration. Compilation of the social security laws—limitations on certain physician referrals. Available at: http://ssa.gov/OP_Home/ssact/title18/1877.htm. Accessed April 14, 2009.
19. Manchikanti L, McMahon EB. Physician refer thyself: is stark II, phase III the final voyage? Pain Physician. 2007;10(6):725–41.
20. Centers for Medicare and Medicaid Services. EMTALA overview. Available at: http://www.cms.hhs.gov/emtala/. Accessed April 14, 2009.
21. Saks SJ. Call 911: psychiatry and the new Emergency Medical Treatment and Active Labor Act (EMTALA) regulations. J Psychiatry Law 2004;32(4):483–512.
22. Greenberg MA, Pincus HA, Ghinassi FA. Of treatment systems and depression: an overview of quality-improvement opportunities in hospital-based psychiatric care. Harv Rev Psychiatry 2006;14(4):195–203.
23. Render ML, Brungs S, Kotagal U, et al. Evidence-based practice to reduce central line infections. Jt Comm J Qual Patient Saf 2006;32(5):253–60.
24. Bigham MT, Amato R, Bondurrant P, et al. Ventilator-associated pneumonia in the pediatric intensive care unit: characterizing the problem and implementing a sustainable solution. J Pediatr April 2009;154(4):582–7. e2. Epub December 3, 2008.
25. Patel KK, Butler B, Wells KB. What is necessary to transform the quality of mental health care. Health Aff 2006;25(3):681–93.
26. Berwick DM, Nolan TW. Physicians as leaders in improving healthcare: a new series in Annals of Internal Medicine. Ann Intern Med 1998;128:289–92.

27. Berwick DM. A user's manual for the IOM's Quality Chasm report. Health Aff 2002; 21(3):80–90.
28. Plsek PE. Section 1: evidence-based quality improvement. Principles and perspectives. Quality improvement methods in clinical medicine. Pediatrics 1999;103(1):203–14.
29. Juran JM. Juran on leadership for quality: an executive handbook. New York: The Free Press, MacMillan, Inc; 1989.
30. Deming WE. Out of the crisis. Cambridge (MA): Center for Advanced Engineering Study; 1986.
31. Institute of Medicine Committee on Quality in Health Care in America. Crossing the quality chasm: a new health system for the 21st century. Washington, DC: National Academy Press; 2001.
32. Keyser DJ, Houtsinger JK, Watkins K, et al. Applying the institute of medicine quality chasm framework to improving health care for mental and substance use conditions. Psychiatr Clin North Am 2008;31:43–56.
33. Pincus HA, Page AE, Druss B, et al. Can psychiatry cross the quality chasm? Improving the quality of health care for mental health and substance use conditions. Am J Psychiatry 2007;164(5):712–9.
34. Volpp KGM, Grande S. Residents' suggestions for reducing errors in teaching hospitals. N Engl J Med 2003;348:851–5.
35. Nelson EC, Batalden PB, Huber TP, et al. Microsystems in health care: part 1. Learning from high-performing front-line clinical units. Jt Comm J Qual Improv September 2002;28(9):472–97.
36. Quinn JB. Intelligent enterprise: a knowledge and service based paradigm for industry. New York: The Free Press; 1992.
37. Mohr JJ, Barach P, Cravero JP. Microsystems in health care: part 6. Designing patient safety into the microsystem. Jt Comm J Qual Patient Saf 2003;29(8): 401–8.
38. Batalden PB, Nelson EC, Edwards, et al. Microsystems in health care: part 9. Developing small clinical units to attain peak performance. Jt Comm J Qual Patient Saf 2003;29(11):575–85.
39. Batalden PB, Nelson EC, Mohr JJ, et al. Microsystems in health care: part 5. How leaders are leading. Jt Comm J Qual Patient Saf 2003;29(6):297–308.
40. Huber TP, Godfrey MM, Nelson EC, et al. Microsystems in health care: part 8. Developing people and improving work life: what front-line staff told us. Jt Comm J Qual Patient Saf 2003;28(10):512–22.
41. Kosnik LK, Espinosa JA. Microsystems in health care: part 7. The microsystem as a platform for merging strategic planning and operations. Jt Comm J Qual Patient Saf 2003;29(9):452–9.
42. Wasson JH, Godfrey MM, Nelson EC, et al. Microsystems in health care: part 4. Planning patient-centered care. Jt Comm J Qual Patient Saf 2003;29(5):227–37.
43. Godfrey MM, Nelson EC, Wasson JH, et al. Microsystems in health care: part 3. Planning patient-centered services. Jt Comm J Qual Patient Saf 2003;29(4): 159–70.
44. Nelson EC, Batalden PB, Huber TP, et al. Microsystems in health care: part 2. Creating a rich information environment. Jt Comm J Qual Patient Saf 2003; 29(1):5–15.
45. Scholtes PR, Joiner BL, Streibel BJ. The team handbook. 3rd edition. Madison, WI: Joiner/Oriel Inc; 2003.
46. Spath PL. Using failure mode and effects analysis to improve patient safety. AORN J 2003;78(1):16–37.

47. Cohen MR, Senders J, Davis NM. Failure mode and effects analysis: a novel approach to avoiding dangerous medication errors and accidents. Hosp Pharm 1994;29:319–29.
48. Shewhart WA. Economic control of quality of manufactured product. New York: Van Nostrand; 1931.
49. Langley GJ, Nolan KM, Norman CL, et al. The improvement guide: a practical approach to enhancing organizational performance. San Francisco (CA): Jossey-Bass; 1996.

Physician Leadership in Residential Treatment for Children and Adolescents

Christopher Bellonci, MD

KEYWORDS

- Residential treatment • Medical Director • Children
- Adolescents • Psychiatry • Consultation-liaison

HISTORY OF RESIDENTIAL TREATMENT FOR CHILDREN AND ADOLESCENTS IN THE UNITED STATES

The role of residential treatment centers (RTCs) in the mental health services array for youth is the direct result of 3 historic trends.[1] The first trend relates to changes in social welfare policy. Many RTCs began as orphanages in the nineteenth century with little or no physician involvement. In the 1960s, social welfare policies changed, and orphanages fell out of favor in the United States.[2] Many of these former orphanages were left without a clear mission. The second trend in the 1970s and 80s saw mental health policy shift away from institutionalization, and many states closed or significantly shrank their psychiatric hospitals for children.[3] The third trend, starting in the 1980s and continuing ever since has been the skyrocketing use of psychiatric medications for children.[4] Former orphanages started adding clinical services and adapted to meet the needs of children and adolescents with serious emotional and behavioral disorders who were no longer being placed in long-term inpatient settings. These children were increasingly referred to RTCs that were ill equipped and that lacked physician leadership to meet the child's mental health needs.

Child psychiatric practice has evolved over the last 50 years from a focus on psychoanalysis to a focus on the biologic treatment of mental illness. RTCs were first developed in the era of psychoanalytic preeminence. Clinicians hoped and believed that theories from psychoanalysis could be applied to children and adolescents within a therapeutic milieu. Psychoanalytic themes also drove the design of psychiatric

Note: Throughout the text, youth and child are used interchangeably to represent the varied age group that residential treatment centers serve.

Walker, 1968 Central Avenue, Needham, MA 02492, USA

E-mail address: cbellonci@walkerschool.org

Child Adolesc Psychiatric Clin N Am 19 (2010) 21–30

doi:10.1016/j.chc.2009.08.001   childpsych.theclinics.com

1056-4993/09/$ – see front matter © 2010 Elsevier Inc. All rights reserved.

inpatient milieus as discussed by Karl Menninger, MD, in vol. 8 of the *Bulletin of the Menninger Clinic*, 1944:

> *If we can love, this is the touch-stone. This is the key to the therapeutic program of the modern psychiatric hospital; it dominates the behavior of its staff from director down to gardener. To our patient who cannot love, we must say by our actions that we do love him. "You can be angry here if you must be; we know you have had cause. We know you have been wronged. We know you are afraid of your own anger, your own self-punishment—afraid, too, that your anger will arouse our anger and that you will be wronged again and disappointed again and rejected again and driven mad once more. But we are not angry—and you won't be, either, after a while. We are your friends; those about you are all friends; you can relax your defenses and your tensions. As you—and we—come to understand your life better, the warmth of love will begin to replace your present anguish—and you will find yourself getting well."*

Loving milieus were believed to be curative.[5] Providing corrective human experiences were the treatments not only for those that had suffered abuse or neglect but also for all individuals presenting with mental illness. With limits, predictability, and nurturance, children could heal from their psychic wounds.

These theories were the foundation for RTCs that were developed in the mid 1900s. All staff working within the residential milieu were seen as agents of therapeutic change. In *The Other 23 Hours*, Al Treischman and his colleagues describe the critical opportunities for therapeutic growth that occurred outside of the therapy hour.[6] Waking children up and preparing them for school was a therapeutic encounter that focused on the organizational and self-regulatory skills required to wash and dress oneself and prepare for the day's tasks. Child care staff working in RTCs were seen as adjunctive therapists, teaching critical skills and coaching the child toward mental health and recovery and providing a corrective experience from that of their early life. Actively teaching competence was a critical component of the model of treatment, predating modern theories of cognitive behavioral therapy.

The field of child psychiatry has undergone significant transformation, with a growing recognition that children suffer from major mental illnesses and could benefit from psychiatric medications for those conditions. RTCs were in need of psychiatric consultation, and differing models of consultation emerged. Most programs use child psychiatrists as direct service providers to work in clinics within RTCs, with responsibility only for prescribing psychotropic medications without further integration into the administrative and leadership structure. As RTCs have evolved to meet the long-term treatment needs of children and adolescents with severe psychiatric conditions, the role of the physician is expanding, leading to the development of executive positions generally characterized as Medical Director. The American Academy of Child and Adolescent Psychiatry's recently prepared *Principles of Care for Treatment of Children and Adolescents with Mental Illnesses in Residential Treatment Centers* offers specific recommendations for the role of the physician leader:

> *The child and adolescent psychiatrist's role should extend and should include attendance at multidisciplinary team meetings, supervise other direct care personnel, involvement in therapeutic program development, and work with the clinical leadership team in monitoring the quality of care and outcomes provided at the RTC. Only providing medication monitoring and other direct patient service is insufficient.[7]*

CURRENT PRACTICE AND CONTROVERSIES

Modern RTCs have recognized and responded to the changing clinical needs of their population by providing multidisciplinary treatment of intermediate duration and acuity between inpatient and outpatient levels of care. RTCs have become tertiary care mental health settings. Children must "fail-up" to gain access.[8] Typically, children will have had multiple prior hospitalizations, many failed medication trials, and multiple attempts at various psychotherapies and behavioral interventions before referral to the RTC. Youth referred to RTCs are, by definition, treatment resistant. Milieu treatment alone is no longer able to meet the needs of this new generation of children being referred for residential treatment, and RTC administrators have recognized the need for child psychiatric consultation.

RTCs are incorporating best practice principles such as family-driven and youth-guided care, and they are using evidence-based clinical practices.[9] The role of the physician in these programs is evolving, and the physician is increasingly being included in leadership roles within these agencies. Although licensing for most RTCs does not formally require a Medical Director, some agencies find it useful to have a physician serve a role in the administration, providing the RTC leadership counsel on strategic planning, risk management, and emerging and best practices. The model of physician leadership that the author outlines in this paper is not standard or universal. The author believes that this model represents the best practice and is a description of the role that he has been fortunate to create as Medical Director at Walker, a multiservice agency that includes residential services for youth with complex emotional and behavioral disorders.

Optimizing Clinical Outcomes: Direct Service

The first, and perhaps most critical, function that physician leadership can provide is a comprehensive review of the child's and family's strengths and needs. The goal is to create a bio-psycho-social-educational formulation that is capable of explaining the child's maladaptive behavior. The child psychiatrist should be able to write a narrative of the child's experiences and risk and protective factors from conception to the present. This means starting with a family history to identify genetically mediated predispositions to illness. It requires a review of potential intrauterine exposure to toxic substances or maternal illnesses and any documentation about the labor and delivery. Understanding the social milieu that the child was born into and whether and what trauma the child may have suffered is essential. Documentation of developmental milestones and when the referral behavior first became manifest provides additional clues to the child's current functioning.

The physician leader needs to have an active curiosity about the causes of children's behavior. Developing a bio-psycho-social-educational formulation is essential to drive the multidisciplinary treatment plan. The process starts with a review by the physician of all past assessments, discharge summaries, diagnoses, and medication trials before placement. Children referred to RTCs have had many treatment interventions by multiple clinicians in various settings. Documenting the history of the child's past treatment is no easy task, as there will often be no single person—parent, guardian, or physician—who can list all the past clinical interventions and medications that were tried and specify whether they were effective or caused side effects. This initial review of records can take a significant amount of time with some children who present with histories of more placements than their age. Careful and scrupulous review is needed to understand the child's risk and protective factors and how to capitalize on their strengths to mitigate their risks.

As the physician conducts his or her initial psychiatric assessment, the other members of the RTC multidisciplinary team review past records and assess the child through their particular professional lens. Occupational therapists assess the child's motor and sensory systems. Speech and language therapists determine how the child is able to use verbal and nonverbal language to communicate his or her feelings and desires and how well the child can interpret nonverbal cues in the environment. Learning disabilities specialists work to understand the child's cognitive and learning abilities and disabilities and how the child uses these abilities in the classroom. Pediatricians evaluate the child's medical and neurologic contributions to their emotional and behavioral functioning and work with the child psychiatrist on how the behavioral disorders and treatment could affect the child's growth and development.

The physician must collect and interpret significant amount of data and then work with the multidisciplinary team to develop a bio-psycho-social-educational formulation about the child's emotional and behavioral presentation. The physician leader must integrate all the past and new information about the child's strengths and needs to come to a hypothesis about the child's behavior. The physician will then make diagnoses incorporating all the available data that will orient the team toward the goals of treatment. When done well, the reasons for the behavior should become self-evident. The formulation should allow a child's caretaker to understand what it is like to be the child carrying past traumas, present challenges, and encountering daily frustrations, as she or he attempts to negotiate complex academic, social, and familial milieus.

Communication among team members is an essential component of residential treatment. Because all staff within an RTC are part of the team working to habilitate the child, they must work with the same understanding of the origins of the problem and how these issues will be treated. The physician plays a critical role in translating the bio-psycho-social-educational understanding of the child into clear instructions on how to work with that child. The child care staff working most closely with the child can bring back to the team on-going data about the effectiveness of the interventions. Frequent meetings of the team allow for this new data to confirm or refute the initial hypotheses about the child's psychopathology, which will then lead to revision of the treatment plan.

Optimizing Clinical Outcomes: Teaching, Training, Consulting, and Coaching

The technology of an RTC is mediated through its staff. The frontline staff who have the most contact with the youth are the least educated and least trained members of the treatment team. In the author's experience, RTC staff, with starting salaries barely above the living wage, are young men and women with an altruistic desire to help society's most vulnerable youth. Most RTCs require a high school diploma or an equivalent, and some child care staff have a bachelor's degree and work in the RTC in anticipation of going back to school for an advanced degree in a related field. This group possesses significant raw talent, but training and supervision is needed to ensure that its altruism is channeled to help teach children to develop self-regulation skills.

The physician leader in these settings is called upon to teach child care staff theories of development and mental illness and its treatments. Child care staff are with the youth throughout the day and are a source of invaluable data regarding the triggers and stabilizers of a child's behavior. They can also provide critical feedback about the response to therapeutic interventions and any treatment-emergent side effects. Physician leadership is needed to identify what data staff need to collect and how to use the data to inform of any changes that may need to be made to the treatment plan. The physician also models, in his or her interactions with children and families, on how to work with dysregulated and challenging youth and can provide on-site coaching in therapeutic interventions, interpreting the youth's behavior and providing concrete recommendations on how staff should respond.

Community-based, nonmedical RTCs are typically not locked milieus. Staff ensure that the children who are being sent with emotional and behavioral disorders remain safe from their aggressive and self-destructive actions. Most RTCs practice some form of physical restraint, and some also use seclusion as a behavior management technique. These are high-risk interventions meant for use only to prevent imminent harm to self and others.[10] The management of restraint is critical, and physician supervision, monitoring, and training of restraint is essential to ensure that youth and staff do not come to harm. Most programs use one of a number of national behavior management programs, but there is no specific accreditation or licensing of behavior-management models and there is much debate in the field about what is safe and what puts the child at the greatest risk. Physicians are needed to help staff design restraint methods that are as safe as possible for the population being served. Individual youth may need adaptation to the standard restraint method being used, based on their size, weight, or medical condition.

Power struggles and issues of control are significant in these settings, both on the part of youth and staff. Young staff coming into the RTC may become frustrated and disillusioned when their well-meaning offers of support or guidance are rebuffed and met with swears, threats, and aggression. It is critical that the counter-aggression that this can elicit is openly discussed and appropriately channeled from the workplace. Physician leaders must be available to identify when these situations occur and provide supervision, modeling adaptive ways of responding to the youth.

Clinical staff in RTCs are typically social workers. They are responsible for individual therapy, family therapy, liaison work with the school and residential staff, and case management with the parent or guardian, lawyers, and other involved systems. The physician and the social worker are the members of the team who have the most holistic understanding of the youth and family's strengths and needs. Working collaboratively, the psychiatrist and social work clinician monitor and document the child's progress and response to treatment. The social work clinician must be trained in multiple modalities of treatment, including psychodynamic psychotherapy, cognitive behavioral therapy, family therapy, trauma-informed treatment, and attachment therapy. They must also understand systems theory and positive behavioral supports. This is a significant body of knowledge, and physician leaders can provide training and supervision for social work staff to help them acquire the requisite skills to be successful with this challenging population.

Some children in RTCs have been abused and neglected by their parents. Staff can engender hostility toward those that abused these children, and this can lead to practices inconsistent with family-driven care, particularly if the goal is reunification with the parent. Where the risk of counter-aggression is ever present for the child care worker, the risk of overidentifying with the youth and not seeing the parent's strengths is ever present for the clinical staff. Physician leaders can provide supervision and consultation to the clinical staff and help educate them about the impacts of multigenerational cycles of violence, parental mental illness, and substance abuse. By enhancing the understanding of the challenges, strengths, and needs of the parent, the physician can help guide the clinical needs and supports for the family.

RTCs are attractive training sites for students from multiple disciplines, including education, social work, psychology, nursing, behavioral pediatrics, and child psychiatry. They offer trainees a clinical setting, with youth presenting with significant psychopathology in a stable treatment setting. Depending on the trainee's discipline and level of experience, they can be provided with significant responsibility for the care of the child and an opportunity to work closely with a multidisciplinary team for a consistent treatment period. The physician leader will be called upon to provide didactic instruction to trainees on a range of topics, including psychiatric assessment and the role of psychopharmacology and psychotherapies in the treatment of youth. At rounds and clinical treatment meetings, the physician leader has an opportunity to think aloud about the origins of the child's behavioral challenges and their risk and protective factors, and to see how to strengthen and teach effective coping skills.

Child psychiatrists working in RTCs must be familiar with how learning and language disabilities can result in frustration for the child and ultimately lead to behavioral disorders. The physician leader works with the educational staff to determine how best to educate the child presenting with the early onset of major mental illness, dealing with trauma, or struggling with profound developmental and cognitive deficits. Student-to-staff ratios are kept small to provide the individualized educational services and supports these children require, which are outlined in their Individual Educational Plans (IEPs). Many of the children in RTCs have a diagnosed learning disability, and teachers need special education training. Many of the classrooms are ungraded, with a wide range of cognitive and developmental abilities, even for children close in age requiring significant academic accommodations.

Teaching staff are typically supplemented with some form of child behavioral specialist and/or teaching assistant in the classroom. These teams must fluidly address the complex mix of learning, emotional, and behavioral needs of the children in their classroom. They must meet the same state-wide curriculum frameworks as public schools. They must also work to maintain a teaching environment for the group while addressing individual children's behavioral outbursts. They are a critical part of the overall team and work closely with the social work case managers and residential staff in developing and applying behavioral plans that are consistent across the various parts of the youth's day. They wear many hats—special educator, behaviorist, and counselor—and often for significantly less pay than that offered in public schools.

Many children in RTCs come with significant developmental challenges and delays. They may have multiple neurodevelopmental deficits that underlie their emotional and behavioral disorders. To assess the youth's strengths and needs and to provide interventions as mandated by their IEPs, RTCs typically employ occupational therapists, speech and language therapists, and physical therapists. These allied health professionals must also be fully integrated into the teams working with each child. For example, best practice would mandate that the child's difficulty with social communication and reading facial expression be seen as essential information not just for the speech and language therapist in pull-out sessions from class but for the entire team working with the child throughout the milieu and to parents at home. As with the physician, it is critical that these allied health professionals be seen as consultants to the team about how the child's individual strengths and needs can be addressed across settings and throughout their day in the milieu. They act as consultants to the child care, educational, and social work staff in the same way the child psychiatrist infuses the team with an understanding of how the child's psychopathology affects their behavior. Their input into the formulation of the child's behavior and the resulting treatment plan is essential.

Family-Driven and Evidence-Based Practice

Historically, many RTCs were suspicious and critical of the role parents played in the origins of their child's psychopathology, and they developed policies and procedures that were hostile to parents. This may have been because of the traditional psychoanalytic view of the origins of mental illness and some of the blaming theories (eg, role of "refrigerator mothers" in schizophrenia) that predominated in the 1950s and 1960s when RTCs were first developing. It may also have been because children were predominantly from the child welfare system, where parents' rights may have been terminated because of abuse and neglect.

Best practice principles view parents and guardians as essential members of the child's treatment team. As such, they drive the child's treatment, with residential staff acting as consultants to the family. All interventions provided by the team should ultimately be focused on helping the child to function in safer and more appropriate ways in the home and community. This requires a clear focus on goals, and any interventions being used in the RTC should be replicable in the home and community setting. Otherwise, children may improve their behavior in the RTC but once discharged, will resume their preadmission maladaptive behaviors. Teaching the skills necessary to parent the child means ensuring that parents and guardians understand the bio-psycho-social-educational formulation that has been developed, agree that it is the best representation of their child's strengths and needs, and develop the skills necessary to implement the treatment plan in the home.

This approach increasingly helps RTCs to work fluidly with families in their home and to have parents work alongside staff in the RTC. In this way, the parents are coached on what works and what does not in terms of their child's behavior. This can be some of the most complex and sophisticated work being done in mental health care, and the physician can play a critical role in providing support and supervision for staff working in the unfamiliar and intimate settings of the child's home. This model requires a deep and abiding respect for families, even when they may not have always been able to meet the needs of their child or when they may continue to struggle with their own mental health needs and challenges. Ensuring that families are not pathologized and are welcome members of the treatment team is an important function of the physician leader.

Emerging practices have RTCs serving as a base for clinical teams that can work with the child and family regardless of the setting. When the child's behavior is more acute and in need of out-of-home stabilization, they might be admitted to the RTC, but once their behavior is stabilized, the same clinical and child care team continues to work with the family in the home, community, and public school setting. The RTC becomes the platform on which community-based care is provided and can be used for brief periods of out-of-home placement as needed. Evidence-based clinical interventions initiated in the RTC could be continued in the outpatient setting by the same team that was working with the child and family. Understanding that mental illness is often chronic and characterized by remissions and exacerbations, this emerging model of care supports continuity between the treatment team and child/family while ensuring that the child is kept safe and in the least-restrictive setting that their emotional and behavioral functioning will allow.

Monitoring of individual progress is critical to inform the interventions being used with the child and family. The physician leader may be called on to help design and implement data collection systems that can monitor and document the progress that a youth is making toward his or her individualized goals. In this way, the team can design a treatment plan with the specificity and measurability of an IEP but with a focus on the child's social, emotional, and behavioral functioning. This can serve as the road map for the child's treatment during and after their residential stay.

Controversies and Critiques of Residential Treatment

RTCs role in the mental health service array has not been without its critics and controversy. The Surgeon General's report on Children's Mental Health highlighted the fact that a quarter of the federal resources that fund children's mental health services go to residential treatment (half is spent on inpatient treatment, and only a quarter on outpatient treatment).[11] This is despite the lack of research showing long-term benefit from residential treatment (also a criticism of inpatient treatment). RTCs generally show improvement in emotional and behavioral functioning of youth from admission to discharge but have less rigorous outcomes when those studies included 1- to 2-year post-discharge follow-up. Defenders of residential treatment will point to the paucity of studies with sufficient scientific rigor to be able to determine the long-term benefits of residential treatment and the difficulty in finding appropriate control groups. They also argue that they cannot be held responsible for outcomes after the child leaves their facility, as they have no control over whether aftercare recommendations are followed, which could result in the child failing to sustain or make anticipated gains.

Some of the criticism of residential treatment focuses on the risks associated with housing youth with similar behavioral disorders in the same setting. The concern is that similar to incarcerated populations, one runs the risk of youth teaching one another how to become more skilled in their sociopathy. However, negative outcomes were more closely related to a lack of active treatment and programming for youth and insufficient training of staff. In programs that included active teaching of skills related to affect management and social problem solving and more rigorous training of staff, worsening sociopathy was not observed. Programming and clinical treatment is critical so that youth are not merely being housed until some date at which they are discharged or aged out of the system.[12]

Unifying Theories of Treatment

The clinical model of residential treatment is about teaching competency and not about cure. When working with a treatment-resistant population, cure is an unreasonable and illusory goal. What is needed is an understanding, via the bio-psycho-social-educational formulation, of what coping skills the child and those working with the child need to learn to function in more adaptive ways, given their social, emotional, and developmental challenges. In essence, the clinical model described in this article teaches skills to the child and to the caretakers (residential and familial). This is slow, and at times, painstaking work that requires a willingness to be patient and to measure success in small increments. Not every physician is suited for this type of work. Understanding one's own professional personality and needs is critical for understanding whether this is the right work setting.

The physician leader in an RTC is the professional with the most extensive mental health training regarding diagnosis and psychiatric care. Working with the other clinical staff, the physician provides the residential program with emerging theories of mental illness and best practices to treat those conditions. It is critical that the physician leader remains current in emerging treatments, both pharmacologic and nonpharmacologic, and be able to impart the new knowledge to others, including those with little or no professional education and training (including parents). This requires the ability to translate complex concepts into simple, nonmedical terms and to make practical recommendations of how to apply the clinical understanding of the child into everyday encounters.

Physician leadership is needed to help RTCs understand their limits of care and remain true to their treatment philosophy. Agreeing to admit and treat a child whose needs go beyond the program's abilities or models of treatment can harm the child, the staff, and the program. Defining which children benefit from residential treatment and why is a critical leadership function. The physician can work with the administration to develop clear admission and discharge criteria. The physician should provide consultation to the admissions staff regarding prospective referrals to the RTC to ensure they meet admission criteria. Physician leaders within RTCs can help to develop outcome studies that can be used to understand better what aspects of the RTC experience account for improvement and which youth benefit most from stays in RTCs. This can be used by the field staff to understand better when and how an RTC stay is appropriate for a specific youth.

Frequently, the physician will be tasked with ensuring that the program's policies and practices are appropriate to ensure that clients and staff do not come to harm. This may include an administrative function of developing and reviewing policies and procedures of the agency, particularly those pertaining to clinical and medical services and behavior management. Working with other administrative leaders and the board of directors, the physician leader can be a valuable resource in the development of the mission, vision, and values of the agency.

Physicians working within the RTCs may be challenged by some continuing hostility to a medical model of care. It is critical that the physician be comfortable with true collaboration, respecting and engaging the other members of the multidisciplinary team as equals, with valuable insights to share about the strengths and needs of the child. A rewarding aspect of this multidisciplinary work is the opportunity to move away from a medical approach defined by a problem list to one that truly works to understand a child's strengths and the ways in which those strengths can be capitalized on to promote healthy, adaptive functioning. The physician can provide a critical synthesizing function as the team develops their bio-psycho-social-educational formulation. In this way, physicians are one among a team of knowledgeable professionals working to promote health and wellness.

It is not uncommon for the physician leader to be the only physician working in an RTC. This can be professionally isolating, and it is important to have access to professional development opportunities with other physicians outside of the RTC and with other physicians working in RTCs. Beyond staying current with emerging practices, it is helpful to have colleagues who can support the challenge of working in a unique, nonmedical clinical setting. There may be no other physician to provide clinical supervision at the RTC, and to ensure that one is aware of clinical "blind spots," supervision with another physician outside of the RTC is recommended. Some physicians seek an academic appointment at a local teaching hospital or medical school as a way of addressing this need. Such an affiliation can also introduce psychiatric trainees to work within an RTC ensuring a future generation of physician leadership for RTCs.

The role of physician leadership within RTCs has paralleled the evolving role of RTCs in the mental health service array for youth. At their best, RTCs provide essential long-term treatment for children with major emotional and behavioral disorders. As the field continues to debate the best ways of providing treatment in the least restrictive setting for children with major mental illnesses, physician leadership will be needed to ensure that this critical part of the service array remains a treatment option.

REFERENCES

1. American Association of Children's Residential Centers. Redefining the role of residential treatment, first in a series of position papers. Available at: http://www. aacrc-dc.org/content/aacrc_position_paper_first_series. Accessed March 6, 2009.
2. Shealy CN. From boys town to Oliver twist, separating fact from fiction in welfare reform and out-of-home placement of children and youth. Am Psychol 1995;50(8): 565–80.

3. Leichtman M. Residential treatment of children and adolescents: past, present, and future. Am J Orthop 2006;76(3):285–94.
4. Olfson M, Marcus SC, Weissman MM, et al. National trends in the use of psychotropic medications in children. J Am Acad Child Adolesc Psychiatry 2002;41(5):514–21.
5. Redl F. The concept of a therapeutic milieu. Am J Orthop 1959;29:721–36.
6. Trieschman AE, Whittaker JK, Brendtro LK. The other 23 hours. Chicago: Aldine Publishing; 1969.
7. Principles of care for treatment of children and adolescents with mental illnesses in residential treatment centers. J Am Acad Child Adolesc Psychiatry 2009, in press.
8. Stuck EN, Small RW, Ainsworth F. Questioning the continuum of care: toward a reconceptualization of child welfare services. Residential treatment for children and youth. vol. 17. 2000. p. 72–92.
9. Lieberman RE. Future directions in residential treatment. Child Adolesc Psychiatr Clin N Am 2004;13:279–94.
10. Masters KJ, Bellonci C, The Work Group on Quality Issues. Practice parameter for the prevention and management of aggressive behavior in child and adolescent psychiatric institutions with special reference to seclusion and restraint. J Am Acad Child Adolesc Psychiatry 2002;41(Suppl 2):4S–22S.
11. US Dept. of Health and Human Services. Mental health: a report of the surgeon general. 1999. Available at: http://www.surgeongeneral.gov/library/mentalhealth/home.html. Accessed March 6, 2009.
12. Dodge KA, Lansford JE, Dishion TJ, editors. Deviant peer influences in programs for youth. New York: Guilford; 2006. p. 3–13.

Directing Child and Adolescent Psychiatry Training for Residents

Sandra B. Sexson, MD

KEYWORDS

- Administration • Child and adolescent psychiatry • Education
- Residents • Medical students

Along with clinical and research agendas, psychiatric education, at the undergraduate and postgraduate levels, is central to the tripartite mission of any academic division of child and adolescent psychiatry (CAP), like that of any department of psychiatry.[1] One could argue that the primary agenda within a school of medicine might well be the educational mission, although it has long appeared to be an underfunded mandate. In CAP within the department of psychiatry, the educational mission may find itself in an even more challenging position, and the child and adolescent psychiatrist who chooses to take on the role as an educational administrator in residency education will find the work complex and challenging: replete with exceptional rewards but fraught with all the difficulties of middle management; one that, to be executed well, must be carried out with much authority, but one that frequently is complicated by being a position with little power. Therefore the administrative aspects of the position require a great deal of interpersonal relationship building and maintenance, along with exceptional administrative skills.

The role of the CAP residency program director (PD) must incorporate the various roles of psychiatric administrators defined in the literature, typically as leadership, administration, and management (**Table 1**).[2–4] The leadership role implies the responsibility to develop a vision and a culture within the training program, the division of CAP and the department of psychiatry that facilitates the program's development of its own unique philosophy and identity beyond the basic standards, its own "brand" of CAP that attracts trainees of similar interest, and an environment in which there is a constant dedication to growth and advancement communicating the strongest commitment to the education of highly competent future child and adolescent psychiatrists. As administrator the major responsibility of the PD is ensuring that the program is in compliance with the standards and requirements established by the Accreditation Council of Graduate Medical Education (ACGME), the Psychiatry Residency Review Committee (RRC), and the local departmental resources and graduate medical

Division of Child, Adolescent and Family Psychiatry, Department of Psychiatry and Health Behavior, Medical College of Georgia, 997 Saint Sebastian Way, Augusta, GA 30907, USA
E-mail address: ssexson@mcg.edu

Child Adolesc Psychiatric Clin N Am 19 (2010) 31–46
doi:10.1016/j.chc.2009.08.010
1056-4993/09/$ – see front matter © 2010 Published by Elsevier Inc.

childpsych.theclinics.com

Table 1
Primary roles of the CAP PD

Leader	Administrator	Manager
Develop a vision for the program	Compliance with requirements	Day-to-day management
Establish critical relationships to facilitate the function of the PD	ACGME:	Work closely with residency coordinator
Department of Psychiatry	Know the requirements	Set up annual calendar in detail and follow it closely
Chair	Follow them as exactly as possible in your program	Use Resident Education Committee as means to develop culture and achieve consensus to promote training issues
Division Chief	Do not ad lib	
Faculty	Keep your documentation up to date; always have a PIF in progress	Delegate responsibilities through committee structure to keep faculty and residents involved and to give yourself more time to deal with the "bigger picture"
Residents	Use the requirements to access the resources you need	
Beyond the department	ABPN:	
Department of Pediatrics	Know the individual requirements	Pay close attention to residency and faculty morale, residency class culture, and support activities that bring fun and education into the program
Neurology	Access sample letters and use them to avoid problems	
Developmental Pediatrics	Always ask if there is a potential credentialing question before you take a resident, not at the end of training. Clarify any questions proactively to protect the individual resident	
Consultation/liaison function		
GME office		
Hospital Administration		
Community mental health		

education (GME) guidelines. Finally, the PD as manager must take care of the day-to-day running of the training program. The CAP PD must balance the need to be obsessive about details of requirements and documentation with flexibility and creativity in finding the best learning opportunities for trainees for various requirements; the need to combine the role of the stern supervisor, when necessary, with that of the available and supportive advocate for the resident; the person who operates the schedule, prompts the tardy evaluations, and so forth, while being the supportive colleague who engages faculty and residents and communicates their value; the "cheerleader," the person who can nurture faculty and residents alike to promote a collective vision, shared successes, and a sense of education as a valued priority. A top-down administrative style is probably not going to work in residency education because teaching, although valued in the academic setting, remains less prestigious than research and less well reimbursed than patient care. Even when faculty members are told that they must teach by the division chief or the chair, their optimal contributions may depend on their active participation and collaboration in the process of the organizational decision making. Bienenfield[5] maintains that the participatory model of administration is particularly advantageous in residency education because it brings the faculty together, engenders more cooperation and ownership of the program and product, helps identify particular skills and interests within the faculty, and improves morale within the faculty even when total unanimity may not be achieved. The PD brings together many players, serving, as Stubbe and colleagues[6] (p 249) suggest to "conduct the symphony," "...transmitting a serious and passionate commitment to the highest standards of comprehensive care for children, adolescents and families, a dedication to residents' personal and professional growth and a vision of the field, where it is and where it needs to go." The symphony often represents, however, a conglomeration of "players" (multiple systems, faculty, trainees, and administrators), who, without the expert orchestration of the administrative skills of the PD, will produce a cacophony of sound rather than the symphonic production of an excellent training program in CAP. This article provides an overview of the key administrative roles of the CAP PD, identifies administrative challenges, and proposes ways to approach achieving the harmonious orchestration that a well-administered training program can produce. When it all works successfully, no position can be more rewarding.

PD, KNOW THYSELF

The person who decides to take on the position of director of training or PD in CAP is assuming a position with many responsibilities and complex interactions. It may seem that the job is straightforward: arranging rotations as prescribed by the ACGME, setting up didactic offerings to meet those requirements, recruiting residents, monitoring and evaluating resident progress and, in general, just doing the same thing year after year. Many division chiefs and department heads fail to recognize the complexity of the position, and many who take on the position do not realize until they are well into feeling overwhelmed that there is much more to administering a good training program than providing the organizational structure for didactics and clinical rotations. This disconnect probably explains why there continues to be such a high turnover rate in the position of PD in our training programs. It behooves anyone considering such a position to make an effort at the beginning to maintain their self-awareness and keep focused on what is meaningful for the training program despite the many distractions that will occur along the way, whether the chief's concern is that everyone's CHILD PRITE (in-training examination) scores are above the 90th percentile versus your concern that your residents are getting experiences that expose them to all of the content that is included on the CHILD PRITE, or whether the clinical service chief needs more residents on the inpatient service while their training needs are for more outpatient experience. Negotiating the environment in which the program occurs requires administrative and leadership abilities that depend on self-awareness[7] and an ability to stay grounded and stick to the things that are important despite external pressures that seem important as well. Even before taking on the position, one should seek out a mentor by talking to another CAP PD. If one is not readily available, one can be accessed by contacting the office of the American Association of Directors of Psychiatric Residency Training (AADPRT) and requesting one through the CAP Caucus. Once one takes the position, many resources are available to the new or seasoned PD (**Box 1**). AADPRT and the American Academy of Child and Adolescent Psychiatry's (AACAP) Work Group on Training and Education provide PDs with a plethora of resources and real-time answers to questions through listservs. No PD should ever believe that there is any administrative question that cannot be posed to these groups for response through their respective listservs. Such support and collegial interaction is invaluable to the work of the CAP PD.

ESTABLISHING THE ENVIRONMENT

The environment in which CAP training occurs is challenging administratively, a fact that is reflected in other sections of this volume and one that has frequently been documented.[2,3,8,9] CAP services are often difficult to sustain financially, and CAP faculties are in short supply. Training and service demands often collide. The PD must be a strong advocate for excellence in training but, to be effective, in doing so must be positioned within the division, the department, the institution, and its administration visibly as one who is a team player committed to the mission of the academic and fiscal functions of the institution overall. Establishing close relationships at all levels within the system in which training will occur is critical for any director of training, but particularly for the CAP PD.

The Department of Psychiatry

Within the department, the CAP PD must be seen as an integral part of the team, not as someone outside the system. The PD must be involved in mainstream departmental administrative activities, because many decisions can have unintended consequences to CAP training. Having CAP training seen as an integral part of departmental functioning keeps CAP educational issues "on the table" and allows the CAP PD to be seen as a major contributor to the overall functioning of the department and not just someone who comes with complaints or requests. A seat on the general psychiatry residency education committee and residency selection committee is invaluable in the overall contributions to education in the department, and in long-term investment in influencing recruitment into the program of residents who may be interested in CAP, and facilitating early and meaningful CAP educational experiences in the training of psychiatry residents to encourage their entry into CAP as well.

The Chair or Chief

Establishing a close relationship with the chair of the department and, of course, with the division chief, is also of the utmost importance, because it is only through these avenues that the ultimate power afforded the PD is assigned and the funding and other resources are allocated. Without the well-established and highly visible support of the department chair and the division chief, the job of the PD is administratively

| Box 1 |
| Resource list |

AADPRT. Every PD should be a member of AADPRT. This organization is your resource for information, for curriculum ideas, for help with challenges, and for anything about training. The organization has a child caucus that specifically addresses CAP issues, although many of the general issues are applicable as well.

Go to Web site http://AADPRT.org to find instructions for joining the organization.

Email: aadprt@verizon.net

Also on the Web site

The newly adopted Common Child and Adolescent Psychiatry Application Form is available at: http://aadprt.org/training/forms/CAP_Common_Application_6-01-09-final.pdf

Numerous training resources; visit the virtual training office

This contains almost anything you want.

Information on GME funding is available at: http://aadprt.org/training/GME/default.aspx

Dictionary of acronyms included in the AADPRT Manual is included here

Information about upcoming and previous meetings

Join the Listserve

The listserve gives you access to many archived discussions and an open forum with current training directors about any question you might pose.

To join the listserve go to the following link: http://www.aadprt.org/members/listserv.aspx and follow the instructions.

AACAP Work Group on Training and Education

Provides links to various resources and an up-to-date list of awards and fellowships available to medical students, psychiatry residents, and CAP residents

Information for medical students and residents: http://www.aacap.org/cs/students.residents.ecp

Information for PDs: http://www.aacap.org/cs/root/physicians_and_allied_professionals/training_and_education

ACGME: http://www.acgme.org is the Web site for all general information concerning the ACGME. For specific information regarding psychiatry, go to the Psychiatry Review Committee site where updates are added frequently.

Current CAP requirements are available at http://www.acgme.or http://www.nrmp.org/fellow/index.htmlg/acWebsite/downloads/RRC_progReq/405pr07012007.pdf

The Chair of the RRC and staff attend AADPRT and present updates at a plenary workshop annually, and also offer 15-minute consultations during the meeting for PDs who have specific questions.

American Board of Psychiatry and Neurology (ABPN): http://www.abpn.com is the Web site for all general information concerning the ABPN. For PDs in CAP the direct link is http://www.abpn.com/cap.htm and more information can be found at http://www.abpn.com/training_programs.htm

The President and Chief Executive Officer (CEO) of the ABPN, along with at least 1 director, and staff members attend the annual AADPRT meeting and present updates at a plenary workshop, and usually offer other workshops as well.

CHILD PRITE: most programs use the CHILD PRITE as the annual cognitive examination required by the ACGME annually for trainees. It is available from the American College of Psychiatrists at http://www.acpsych.org or, more specifically, at http://www.acpsych.org/prite/pritedates.html

National Residency Matching Program (NRMP): The ACGME in its Institutional Requirements states that programs "should" participate in match programs when they are available. CAP has had a match through NRMP since 1995. This program can be accessed through the Web site at http://www.nrmp.org or, more specifically, on the fellowship page at http://www.nrmp.org/fellow/index.html.

MedEdPortal: an Association of American Medical Colleges (AAMC) online peer reviewed service that collects teaching and assessment tools and other faculty development resources. It houses a psychiatry medical student collection. It is a place where psychiatric educators can publish their curricular projects. It can be accessed at http://services.aamc.org/30/mededportal/servlet/segment/mededportal/information/.

impossible. In small programs, often the division chief may also serve as the PD, making the relationship with the department chair even more critical.

The faculty

As noted earlier, the PD is a middle manger, and therefore must maintain close leadership roles with the faculty to facilitate an optimal educational environment for the training program. Establishing a good working relationship with the faculty is an ongoing endeavor that requires continuous nurturing, intensive monitoring, and focused efforts to discern faculty strengths and organize the teaching and supervisory efforts of each faculty member to play to the person's strengths and interests to optimize their successes as educators. As a PD, I have found that establishing what each faculty member most enjoys doing, teaching, supervising, and being sure that his/her particular assignment reflects those interests is the best recipe for success, even if it means that I often find myself teaching different things from year to year because I eventually may be the one "filling in the holes" where there is little interest or enthusiasm. In the long run, having excited and motivated teachers is a major part of creating a positive learning environment. The PD must find ways to let faculty know when they are doing a good job, even in small ways that may, on the surface, seem insignificant: a brief email with a copy to the chief or the chair, a "good job" sticker (after all, this is *child* psychiatry), verbal praise at a faculty meeting, and so forth, in addition to teaching awards, facilitation of local and national awards, committee appointments, travel funding, and the like. Involving everyone in the process of training, in the ongoing planning of educational growth and changes, in making the program "ours" as opposed to "mine" or that of a few of the leaders, all of these efforts facilitate better faculty involvement and greater contributions. It also makes it more fun for the PD as well. A recent article suggests that dividing the responsibilities for many of the administrative tasks of the PD within a training program among the faculty may actually free up some of the administrative time of the PD to allow for more time for working on the vision, while also improving efficiency and output from the various faculty members of the residency education committee.[10] Another way to engage faculty is to encourage academic development through educational research or publications regarding curricular development on peer reviewed Web sites such as MedEdPortal.

The residents

Although the PD must establish critical relationships within the department with the leadership and with the faculty, he/she must also establish a complex relationship with the residents.[2] PDs serve many roles to residents as outlined by Beresin,[2] shifting from one to the other seamlessly most of the time, sometimes not recognizing which one until a resident points it out as one of mine did recently: when I encouraged her again to get something done, she responded to my email with a "Yes, mother." Most PDs don't pay much attention to these roles until there is a problem with a resident, and then it becomes an issue, but it is important to constantly take stock of the relationships, to recognize the dynamic processes that are constantly in play with the individual relationships and with the group of residents as a whole, and to maintain a relationship that allows a comfort and safeness and that facilitates the expression of vulnerability as necessary, while retaining the ability to exert authority, discipline, and appropriate guidance and remediation when appropriate. This empathic balance requires a strong sense of boundaries and an attention to developing opportunities to interact with all residents in multiple clinical and academic settings throughout their training, creating an atmosphere in which all residents believe that their PD values them as individuals and serves as an advocate for their education and their professional development fairly and equally.

Beyond the Department of Psychiatry

The child and adolescent PD must not limit his/her sphere of influence to the Department of Psychiatry but must also develop relationships within the Department of Pediatrics. First, developing strong pediatric ties is important for certain clinical experiences such as pediatric consultation/liaison, neurology, and developmental disabilities. Often, support from pediatrics is also critical to survival in hospital settings. In addition, finding contributory medical staff roles in hospital administration and in the academic practice plan allows the CAP PD to maintain a presence at an institutional level that can be helpful when administrative challenges arise. Maintaining these relationships across the medical school environment is critical for the CAP PD who wants to be seen as part of the administrative team and not as a misunderstood outsider. Beyond the institution, depending on the particular training program, the PD may also need to establish relationships with community agencies, state systems, and other mental health (MH) providers to facilitate development of training opportunities. The possibilities are always expanding and the wise PD is constantly on the lookout for new opportunities for creative educational experiences and funding options for training in CAP.

Finally good working relationships must be established with the local GME office, the GME committee, the designated institutional officer (DIO) and the office's various administrative assistants. Although CAP is not considered strictly as a subspecialty of psychiatry by the ACGME, one often has to ensure that CAP gets adequate attention in the local GME office, especially in relation to funding issues. Funding is a major issue for CAP PDs because not all of the funding lines available to psychiatry programs are readily available to CAP programs. CAP PDs need to understand GME funding sources at a national and a local level, and work closely with their GME office and within their own division and department to assure adequate funding for their resident stipends.[11] Serving on GME committees, ad hoc review committees, and, again, becoming a known entity in the local GME administrative structure is an important aspect of making sure that the CAP PD remains involved in critical GME decision-making circles at the local institutional level.

THE ADMINISTRATIVE FUNCTIONS
The Leadership Role

This article identifies the 3 major roles of the psychiatric administrator (see earlier discussion). Much of what has been discussed (ie, the establishment of the many relationships that create the setting for the successful CAP training program) may be subsumed ultimately within the leadership role, for much of this is involved in looking to the future, developing a vision, and setting a standard for training that is above and beyond what is adequate or basic. The PD must lead the faculty and each residency group to find better ways to address acquisition and measurement of competencies in CAP. I am often asked during recruitment season how certain things are done in our program, I find myself frequently commenting that this is the way it is done now but, by the time the applicant might join the program, a new and better way might have been found, because a good training program is constantly changing as the vision moves the program forward. It is the leadership of the PD that mobilizes the faculty and the residents to join their resourceful and innovative energies to create a vibrant and ever-evolving program.

Recruitment

It is difficult to decide where to put resident recruitment in the overall administrative structure of the role of the residency PD. Ultimately it is the most important role because, without residents, there is no training program. Recruitment into CAP is a major priority because of the magnitude of the recognized shortage of child and adolescent psychiatrists to meet the projected needs for the treatment of child mental disorders.[12] Yet, as a PD, you have essentially only 1 pipeline from which to recruit trainees: general psychiatry training programs whose numbers have remained stable over the past several decades. New portals for entry into CAP training are being sought. Triple board programs that combine pediatrics, psychiatry, and CAP have been in place for more than 20 years, but it is unclear whether they will expand. These programs recruit residents directly out of medical school. The ACGME is sponsoring a new, innovative, limited pilot-project program called the Post Pediatrics Portal Project (PPPP) in which approved programs take fully trained pediatricians and combine general and child training into a 3-year training period. For information about this potential training opportunity to expand recruitment possibilities, go to http://acgme.org/acWebsite/navPages/nav_400.asp. Aside from this, CAP programs typically recruit from the general psychiatry pool. Currently the Psychiatry RRC, through the Institutional Requirements expects training programs to participate in the National Residency Matching Program (NRMP) in child psychiatry. Information about this program can be found on the NRMP Web site at http://NRMP.org. The match in child psychiatry takes place earlier in the year than the general match, with the rank order list (ROL) deadline usually in early to late December, and match date sometime in mid January for residency start dates the following July. Therefore most programs start accepting resident applications in July and August, and begin their interview seasons in the late summer and early fall. Most PDs plan to recruit from within their own programs by serving on the psychiatry recruitment committee to recruit into psychiatry medical students who are already interested in CAP, and then work with the CAP faculty to nurture this interest and to pique the interest in CAP of other psychiatry residents in training. Thus much recruitment effort is at the local level. However, most programs will also want to recruit candidates from outside their programs. The PD must use public relations (PR) skills, including Web site expertise, to highlight the brand that makes the local program unique and inviting for the right resident fit, and then must orchestrate an interview experience that gives the PD and faculty a chance to evaluate the applicant, but also provides an opportunity to "sell" the program, because the recruitment process is definitely a "buyer's" market. Involving your most excited residents and faculty in the applicant interview process, finding out some of the special interests of the applicants before they come and pairing them with those who have common interests locally, and carefully planning follow-up contacts are key strategies for successful recruitment. Recruiting the highest-quality residents with the best fit for your particular training program is the most important responsibility of the PD. The rules of the match prohibit the PD from basing any expression of interest in a candidate on the candidate's willingness to commit to the program. However, if the PD is going to rank the candidate high enough to match in the program, the PD can indicate this to a highly desirable candidate. New PDs are often disappointed when match results come out and they find that applicants they believed were coming to their programs did not match with their program. Applicants learn to keep their options open, so it is always best to base your ROLs on who you think are the best candidates for your program, and not necessarily on who you think is most likely to rank you first. Seasoned PDs will frequently tell you that those latter assumptions are often disappointing. One of the details on which every PD must concentrate is to remind all applicants to turn in their ROL and to check that their own is correctly submitted and documented on the NRMP Web site. Too many candidates and programs have been disappointed because of mistakes at this level of functioning (**Box 2**).

The Administrative Role

The ACGME

The administrative role of the PD is to assure that the program is in compliance with the ACGME Program Requirements for Training in CAP, which can be accessed at the ACGME Web site on the Psychiatry RRC page (http://www.acgme.org/ac

---

Box 2
Tips for recruiting

1. Establish a brand and vision for your program, and communicate it well on your Web site and in your brochure, if you develop one. Also remember that recruiting happens throughout the year wherever you, your faculty, your chair, and your chief come into contact with other faculty and psychiatry residents and medical students. Getting your program known, so that applicants will consider looking at it when recruitment time comes, is the first step to recruiting someone to your program.

2. Begin planning your recruitment season in late spring, setting up interview schedules with selected residents and faculty, facility tours, and recruitment packages that give information about your program and your community. Remember that you are in the PR and selling mode. You want everyone you interview to WANT to come to your program. Then you have choices.

3. Respond to inquiries about your program in a timely manner with good information about your process and timing for interviews.

4. Be sure that every interview day is well planned, and avoid glitches if at all possible. Choose your most excited residents and faculty to interview. Arrange to get feedback immediately after the interviews. It is useful for the PD to see the candidates in some venue at the beginning of the day and the end of the day to orient and debrief, if at all possible.

5. Carefully plan follow-up with all candidates, but particularly those whom you really want to recruit. Having one of the residents "touch base" shortly after the visit to field any questions, and then the PD or a faculty member who seemed to hit it off with the candidate touch base a week or so later, is also a good idea.

6. Maintain contact throughout the recruitment season, without being too pushy.

7. Approximately 2 weeks before the ROL is due, email the candidates and express continued interest (if you plan to rank them), and remind them of your NRMP number and the ROL deadline. For those candidates whom you plan to rank high enough that they are sure to match in your program (should they choose to rank you high enough, that is), you could indicate to your top 4 (if you have a complement of 4) that you are ranking them high enough to match with your program. That statement requires no response on their part, but is just a statement of fact. Some PDs choose to do this and others do not, but it is permitted under the Match Agreement. You cannot just promise a match and fail to rank the candidate high enough that he/she will match. You absolutely cannot make such a promise conditional on the applicant committing to ranking you high on their list.

8. After your ROL has been submitted to the NRMP, relax and enjoy the holidays, and go on with other residency training functions. Plan a celebration party for the afternoon of Match Day for those within your program who match into your program and for all those who assisted with the recruitment process. It is a great way to complete the recruitment season. Be sure to make contact with your matched applicants on Match Day to welcome them to your program.

Website/downloads/RRC_progReq/405pr07012007.pdf). These requirements are revised approximately every 5 years. Anyone assuming the position of PD should make it the first priority to read these requirements carefully, especially the specific ones, the common requirements, and the institutional requirements. Some PDs fear the ACGME and its requirements, but often the requirements can be helpful to the PD in getting resources to support adequate training. The Requirements outline not only the clinical experiences that each trainee should have during the training but lists didactic content and schedules for evaluations, structure for oversight, and other administrative requirements. Each program is reviewed by the Psychiatry RRC on a scheduled basis, depending on the length of time allotted at the previous review. Before the review, the program is notified and the PD must prepare a detailed Program Information Form (PIF) that addresses how the particular program is meeting all of the requirements for training. The PIF is provided to the RRC and to the site visitor assigned to visit the program. The site visitor visits the program to ascertain that what is reported in the PIF is what is happening in the program. The site visitor's job is to verify what is reported in the PIF to the RRC, and not to pass judgment on whether the program is meeting the requirements. The RRC members then review the site visitor's report, the PIF of the PD, and the program history available at the ACGME, and make a decision about accreditation or any concerns or citations that need to be addressed. The major administrative role of the PD is to assure that the program is in compliance with the ACGME Requirements. Being sure that you understand each requirement and take each one of them seriously and concretely is absolutely necessary. If the Requirements say that the Program Letter of Agreement with an affiliated training site needs to be renewed every 5 years, then do so even if both parties believe that there have been no changes in the agreement. The RRC requires the renewal. If a requirement says something has to be in writing, you will probably be asked to show the site visitor evidence of the product in writing. When there is specific language in the requirements, it is best to adhere to the language used. For instance, in the section on summative evaluations (V.A.2.b) the Requirements specify that the summative evaluation "must verify that the resident has demonstrated sufficient competence to enter practice without direct supervision."[13] Follow the guidelines verbatim. If there is specific wording, use it. Do not try to be creative or to demonstrate your proficient writing skills. Use your creativity to develop better teaching and evaluation methodologies, to bring together faculty, and to promote enthusiasm, but, when it comes to complying with the details of the RRC Requirements, it is always best to attend specifically to the details and be sure you maintain your compliance as close to the requirement as possible. Adhering to these kinds of specifics requires a thorough knowledge of the Requirements and a commitment to adhering to the details that they contain. Remember that the Review Committee only has the information that you report in your PIF and whatever the site visitor describes, so be sure that you give as much information as possible. Decisions can only be made on the information available. If you have questions about a specific requirement and how it may be met, do not hesitate to ask someone. Ask your PD mentor or go directly to the AADPRT Listserv or the AACAP Training Listserv. However, help is also available at the RRC, and the staff there will answer your questions whenever necessary. Each year at the AADPRT meeting there is a plenary workshop during which the Chair and staff members of the RRC review any changes in the Requirements and are available to answer questions. RRC members and staff usually also offer individual consultation times during the AADPRT meeting in case you have some specific questions that you would like to discuss. Know the Requirements. Be sure that you are integrating them into your program and that you demonstrate how you are doing so when you report to the RRC. And when your site is visited, prepared your PIF carefully, giving accurate and complete information. Involve your faculty and your residents in this preparation, and, before the site visitor comes, be sure that all those who will meet with the surveyor have reviewed the information that has been given to the site visitor and are in agreement with what has been reported. If you correct any discrepancies before the visit you will be prepared (**Box 3**).

The institution's GME office
The PD has other administrative standards to meet for the trainees during the course of their training. Each institution's GME office will have numerous require-ments, many of which reflect the ACGME Institutional Requirements, but some of which stem from state, hospital, or medical school demands. Responding to these demands in a timely manner, volunteering to serve on ad hoc internal review committees, participating in institutional GME activities and retreats; all these activ-ities foster good relationships that support your program through RRC reviews and other stressful times.

The ABPN
The PD also needs to be continually cognizant of the requirements for credentialing to apply for ABPN certification examinations. There is usually coordination between ACGME requirements and ABPN requirements, but ACGME is concerned with programs whereas ABPN is concerned with individual trainees. As a PD, it is your responsibility to assure that each trainee has completed all of the requirements for

---

Box 3
Tips for achieving compliance with the accrediting agencies

1. The ACGME Requirements for Training in Child and Adolescent Psychiatry is your guidebook. Know it from beginning to end, and be sure that your coordinator knows it as well.

2. Emphasize to your faculty the parts of the Requirements that apply to the components of training in which they play roles, and engage their contributions to ongoing compliance.

3. Be sure that the residents are also aware of what they should expect from their training, as defined by the RRC, and what is expected of them as well. Involving the residents as collaborators makes the compliance process easier as well.

4. Address each requirement individually and identify how you are addressing it in your program; document what you are doing and be sure that the documentation that is required is included in the ongoing document that will be your PIF at site visit time.

5. Explore any questions that you have about what a requirement may mean, whether what you have in place will meet the requirement, or what you may need to change to reach compliance. Bring up concerns regularly in your Residency Education Committee, and develop plans to address these concerns proactively. Do not wait until site visit or midcycle review time to address deficiencies or concerns. Keep abreast of any problems and fix them as they develop.

6. Stay informed about ABPN requirements and meet requirements for your residents so that each can be credentialed to be examined for certification at the earliest date possible. This important criterion is one of the assessment factors the RRC uses to evaluate your program, and it is important to your graduates as they move into their practice situations. Again, adhering exactly to the requirement, using their sample letters, and keeping abreast of any changes is imperative.

7. Stay informed. Follow the rules, and then do not worry about the oversight.

being credentialed to be examined for ABPN certification. Particular attention needs to be paid to those trainees who do not do all of their training in your program, but who will complete their training in your program because it will be you who has to ascertain that they have completed the necessary requirements. In CAP, this is more often than not because most of our trainees are credited with their final year of Psychiatry while they are doing their first year of CAP training. It is imperative that you be sure that, at the end of their third year, you have final documentation from the psychiatry PD that they have completed all of their psychiatry-specific requirements so that you can confirm completion of psychiatry training after the first year of CAP training. Again, AADPRT meetings are a good place to meet with the President and CEO and some of the directors and staff of the ABPN and hear about changes that are taking place. Their Web site has a special section for PDs.[14] Sample letters needed to confirm resident's training experiences are available. Again, as before, use these samples verbatim. Do not rephrase. It is much safer to use their wording to avoid problems for you and your residents who are applying to take their board certification examinations. Compliance, not innovation, is the key administrative task in these endeavors. Once you have these documentations organized, they can be routinized into the annual schedules by the program coordinator and become a part of the managing component of training administration.

New requirements

During the past 10 or so years, the ACGME has required the development of specialty-specific competencies which now need to be evaluated. Much has been, and will continue to be, written about the specifics of this, and the wise PD will be looking to his/her colleagues and to AADPRT regularly to continually update the program in these areas.[15] Recently, the ABPN announced that residents beginning training in July 2010 on the traditional track will be required to have successfully completed 3 clinical skills evaluations during training to be eligible to take the examination for certification by ABPN in the subspecialty of CAP. Further information regarding how this requirement must be met may be found at the ABPN Web site at http://www.abpn.com/downloads/forms/ABPN_CSV_form_v2.pdf. In addition, as with any other new challenges, AADPRT and AACAP meetings and Web sites feature ways to meet the requirements for the clinical skills verification (CSV). The CAP PD must always be alert for new requirements, new challenges, and new opportunities because the field is continually evolving.

The Managing Role

The day-to-day administration of the CAP training program requires the ability to see the "big picture," looking always to the future while paying attention to the tedious repetitive details that take place on an annual basis.

The residency coordinator

The fortunate PD works with a talented residency coordinator, a support position required by the ACGME with adequate time to support the residency program.[13] The residency coordinator maintains the residency office, coordinating the primary functions of the office, including recruitment, scheduling, assessment, and record-keeping. In fact, the residency coordinator is usually the first contact that applicants have with the program when they call or email to request information. He or she is also frequently the person to whom residents come first with problems. Personal characteristics that balance warmth and openness with the ability to maintain boundaries and structure are ideal in this position.[5] The coordinator is the "go-to" person for any question about any of the daily functions of the program, and is the person who maintains all the records needed for site visits, graduated residents, faculty teaching activities, and so forth. Coordinators facilitate scheduling of seminars, special activities, and examinations; they solicit timely evaluations, assure resident compliance with local, state, and national GME requirements, and so forth. With the PD they ideally develop an annual calendar that fits their program (**Table 2**) to anticipate these tasks and keep the office on schedule. A good working relationship between them goes a long way toward assuring that the managing role of the PD is achieved successfully.

Teaching, evaluation and, if necessary, remediation
Ultimately the goal of the PD is that of graduating physicians who are committed to, and able to provide, the highest standards of practice in CAP. Much of what the PD orchestrates as experiences for the trainees involves the educational competencies that facilitate the achievement of the ability to practice competently and independently. The content, even the techniques, for evaluation and remediation are addressed in numerous volumes elsewhere in the literature. However, clinical supervisors frequently are unwilling to accurately evaluate residents who are performing poorly.[16] It is important administratively for the PD to recognize the barriers that lead to inaccurate reporting and work with faculty regularly in an attempt to avoid these barriers. Encouraging faculty to keep records of examples of problems during rotations so that, when the time comes to write the evaluation there will be some example to give, is helpful. When a problem arises, helping faculty to specifically document the problem also makes it possible for the PD to better address it with the trainee and work to remediate the issue. Sometimes faculty members are concerned that there will be an appeals process ,and therefore resist expressing negative feedback. Often this occurs because faculty members have felt their own credibility was questioned or they have not been supported when they have expressed concerns in the past, or that supporting their concerns or confronting residents with performance problems requires too much time. Finally, faculty members felt failing a trainee was a problem if remediation was not available or if they did not believe they could help the trainee. All of these potential obstacles to faculty willingness to report concerns about resident performance must be addressed in training programs. It is important for the PD to establish an administrative structure and a culture that supports faculty in expressing concerns about poor performance early and effectively. Individual and group venues in which residents are discussed with the PD may facilitate this process and encourage better assessment techniques and a greater willingness to accurately assess residents. Making it the program's problem to develop a remediation plan, not the responsibility of the individual supervisor, also relieves some of the resistance to reporting problems. It is important to establish in the beginning a culture with residents in which the expectation is that every resident, even the most outstanding, can identify areas where improvements can be made. Encouraging faculty and residents on all evaluation forms to avoid all "outstandings," and to identify strengths, and, if not weaknesses, then "areas to focus on for improvement over the next 3 to 6 months" facilitates much more useful evaluations and more focused individualized learning management plans for each trainee. Having this kind of culture, which looks for areas to improve rather than weaknesses or areas of failure, makes it easier for everyone to embrace the need for change, whether small or more moderate. Developing supervision groups for supervisors in which supervisors get together with an experienced supervisor, may provide a venue where supervisors can discuss the supervisory process and become more comfortable at giving negative feedback formally and informally. As PDs, it is our professional and administrative responsibility

Table 2
CAP PD and coordinator's suggested calendar

July	August	September
Orientation and welcome new residents	Set up recruitment dates with faculty/resident appointment schedules through first week in December	Coordinate with psychiatry program for CAP residents to take PRITE and clear schedules for PRITE
Mail ABPN letters for graduating residents (due July 15)	Begin reviewing applications	Schedule Resident Selection Committee meetings if different from Resident Education Committee
Order CHILD PRITE examinations and set date for examination	AADPRT renewal	Continue recruitment
Schedule semiannual reviews for second year residents		Quarterly evaluations
Review recruitment schedules/materials		AADPRT meeting workshop submissions

October	November	December
PRITE examination	ABPN CAP oral examinations until they are discontinued	CHILD PRITE
AACAP annual meeting (training forum, PD's dinner)	Final arrangements for CHILD PRITE administration	CAP match ROL due
		Holiday party
		Six-month evaluations

January	February	March
Child match results	Plan for mock boards or oral examinations	AADPRT meeting (Child Caucus meetings, RRC and ABPN large workshops, CAP workshops)
Announce match results	Finish preparations for any workshops presenting at AADPRT meeting	Graduation plans
Send appointment letters for newly matched residents		Quarterly evaluations
Schedule and conduct semiannual evaluations for all residents		Oral examinations

April	May	June
Begin rotation/supervision assignments	APA	Graduation
Begin seminar scheduling	Schedule final evaluation meetings	Academic project presentations
Mailings to incoming residents	Graduation planning	Exit procedures
	Order graduation certificates	Final evaluation for graduating residents
	Finalize rotation/supervision assignments	New resident files
	Finalize orientation schedule	Finalize seminar schedules for coming academic year
	Continue seminar scheduling	

to assure that we take seriously the evaluation of our trainees, and have objective and subjective support for the statements we make at the end of training about their competence to practice independently.

What about Medical Students?

Unfortunately few child and adolescent psychiatrists are directors of medical student education in schools of medicine. However, the AACAP is encouraging all divisions of CAP to actively engage medical students regarding issues of child, adolescent, and family mental health. PDs in CAP may be best positioned to work directly with the department's Director of Medical Student Education to ensure that medical students get a chance to see child and adolescent psychiatrists at work. Find opportunities for faculty and residents to teach in the preclinical and clinical years by volunteering to lecture, and teach in interviewing courses and workshops. Lobby for CAP topics in clerkship lecture series. Develop clerkship sites that offer CAP experiences within the medical school and within the community, even if it is only for a week or 2 of the clerkship experience. Also develop M-4 electives that either entirely focus on CAP or include CAP experiences. Enlist the CAP faculty to serve as faculty advisors for medical students or mentor medical students, and be sure the PD and other CAP faculty are involved in the local psychiatry interest groups (PsychSIGN). AACAP (http://AACAP.org) has numerous resources available for medical students that can be accessed to augment efforts to introduce students to the exciting field of CAP.

SUMMARY

The PD in CAP is an administrative position that incorporates all the roles of the psychiatric administrator (those of leader, administrator, and manager) and, in all these roles, the PD is in the position of middle management, constantly being pulled in all directions, working from a position that requires authority but has little power, and thus requiring significant leadership and interpersonal skills. The administrative role demands an attention to the specifics of requirements that is tedious and at times fairly rigid. The PD therefore needs to be flexible and perhaps somewhat of a sales person, and also somewhat of an accountant, crossing the *t*'s, dotting the *i*'s, and being sure that everything is getting done in the proper way at the proper time. The job can be challenging at times, sometimes frustrating, slightly overwhelming, at times repetitive, but usually stimulating, and always gratifying when one sees the product of one's efforts a few years later leading the local chapter of the Academy, assuming a faculty position, recognized as a local community leader, mentioned as someone who was helpful by a grateful patient, or publishing the lead article in a prestigious journal. Also, at the end of each residency year, I usually find myself saying at graduation that we have worked hard to be sure they have been exposed to the best evidence-based treatments, but that most of what has been learned will be out of date within a few years, if not months, from the time they graduated. However, if they have internalized a way to relate well to youth and families, and to colleagues, a commitment to, and love for, lifelong learning, a zeal for constantly looking for better ways of practicing and serving the patients they see, and a professional dedication to their patients that rises above personal needs, then whatever knowledge or clinical skill is necessary will be acquired and our goals of training will definitely have been achieved.

REFERENCES

1. Meyer R. The tripartite mission of an academic psychiatry department and the roles of the chair. Acad Psychiatry 2006;30(4):292–7.

2. Beresin E. The administration of residency training programs. Child Adolesc Psychiatr Clin N Am 2002;11(1):67–89.

3. Cohen R. Developing a functional administrative structure. In: Cohen R, Dulcan MK, editors. Basic handbook of training in child and adolescent psychiatry. Springfield (IL): Charles C Thomas; 1987. p. 213–24.

4. Faulkner L. Development as a psychiatric administrator. In: Kay J, Silberman EK, Pessar LF, editors. Handbook of psychiatric education and faculty development. Washington, DC: American Psychiatric Publishing, Inc; 1999. p. 549–72.

5. Bienenfeld D. Administration of the residency program. In: Kay J, Silberman EK, Pessar LF, editors. Handbook of psychiatric education. Washington, DC: American Psychiatric Press, Inc; 2005. p. 125–42.

6. Stubbe D, Heyneman E, Stock S. A stitch in time saves nine: intervention strategies for the remediation of competency. Child Adolesc Psychiatr Clin N Am 2007;16(1):249–64.

7. George B, Sims P, McLean AN, et al. Discovering your authentic leadership. Harv Bus Rev 2007;1–8.

8. Sexson S. Overview of training in the twenty-first century. Child Adolesc Psychiatr Clin N Am 2007;16(1):1–16.

9. Westman J. Administrative issues in child and adult psychiatry training programs. Child Psychiatry Hum Dev 1978;8(4):195–201.

10. van Zyl LT, Finch S, Davidson PR, et al. Administrative restructuring of a residency training program for improved efficiency and output. Acad Psychiatry 2005;29(5):464–70.

11. Magen J. Psychiatry training: GME funding. Available at: http://www.aadprt.org/training/GME/default.aspx. 2007. Accessed July 26, 2009.

12. AACAP. AACAP workforce fact sheet. Available at: http://www.aacap.org/cs/root/legislative_action/aacap_workforce_fact_sheet. 2009. Accessed July 22, 2009.

13. ACGME. ACGME program requirements for training in child and adolescent psychiatry. Available at: http://www.acgme.org/acWebsite/downloads/RRC-progREQ/405pr/7012007.pdf. Accessed July 22, 2009.

14. ABPN. Residency training programs. Available at: http://abpn.com/training_programs.htm. 2009. Accessed July 22, 2009.

15. Varley C. Training. In: Martin A, editor, Child and adolescent psychiatric clinics of North America, vol. 16. Philadelphia: Elsevier, Inc; 2007. p. 270.

16. Dudek NL, Marks M, Regehr G. Failure to fail: the perspectives of clinical supervisors. Acad Med 2005;80(10):S84–7.

Child and Adolescent Psychiatry Leadership in Public Mental Health, Child Welfare, and Developmental Disabilities Agencies

Albert A. Zachik, MD[a,*], Michael W. Naylor, MD[b,c], Robert L. Klaehn, MD[d,e]

KEYWORDS

- Child and adolescent mental health • Child welfare
- Developmental disabilities • Child psychiatry administration
- Systems of care

A child and adolescent psychiatrist working as a lead administrator in the public mental health system is in a unique position to assist children, youth, and families because of their special training. Unique to the training of a child and adolescent psychiatrist is the in-depth understanding of the dynamics that influence large systems of care. Child psychiatrists are taught to work within a family system respecting the knowledge, opinions, and culture of parents and caregivers to inform about the young person being evaluated and treated. With that as a base the public mental health administrator must understand and work within systems that include other health care providers, state education systems, child welfare, juvenile justice, developmental disabilities, and substance abuse services. Consultation to and with others is a major part of training. Group therapy skills hone the ability to understand the dynamics within group process, to understand other's opinions, viewpoints, and perspectives, improving the ability to

[a] State of Maryland Department of Health and Mental Hygiene, Mental Hygiene Administration, Office of Child and Adolescent Services, Spring Grove Hospital Center, Dix Building, 55 Wade Avenue, Catonsville, MD 21228, USA
[b] Department of Psychiatry, University of Illinois, Chicago, IL 60608, USA
[c] Behavioral Health and Welfare Program, Institute for Juvenile Research, Room 155, 1747 West Roosevelt Road, M/C 747, Chicago, IL 60608, USA
[d] Arizona Division of Developmental Disabilities, Arizona Department of Economic Security, 1789 West Jefferson, Site Code 791A, Phoenix, AZ 85007, USA
[e] Maricopa Integrated Health System Child Psychiatry Residency Program, AZ, USA
* Corresponding author.
E-mail address: azachik@dhmh.state.md.us (A.A. Zachik).

Child Adolesc Psychiatric Clin N Am 19 (2010) 47–61
doi:10.1016/j.chc.2009.08.007
childpsych.theclinics.com
1056-4993/09/$ – see front matter © 2010 Elsevier Inc. All rights reserved.

work with others. In addition, the child and adolescent psychiatrist working within large public systems must use their full understanding of the range of treatment modalities along the continuum for outpatient services, including wraparound and home-based services to inpatient and residential treatment.

Working within a state mental health agency, a child psychiatrist uses all of these skill sets in his or her work with both individual patients and their families but also with broad and diverse populations. A major part of the work is to plan for mental health services for children and youth and supports for their families and caregivers in many settings. These settings include early childhood screening and intervention programs, school-based mental health programs, child welfare foster care settings and group homes, and juvenile justice detention centers. The services include an array from more intense inpatient hospital and residential treatment settings, to wraparound home- and community-based services including afterschool treatment or rehabilitation programs; respite care; mentoring; mobile treatment and crisis response; in-home stabilization systems; and the traditional outpatient treatments of individual, family, and group therapies.

On a systems level the child mental health director works to identify what types of treatment and interventions a community might need; works with legislators and the executive branch of their states to make funds available to develop appropriate early identification, assessment, and treatment programs; takes the lead in designing and implementing these programs; and monitors their quality and effectiveness. On an individual level the child mental health director is called on to review the appropriateness and availability of care for specific children who might not easily fit into a pre-existing program.

Each state and system work independently to meet the mental health needs of its residents. Given the extraordinary cultural and ethnic diversity of the country the needs of residents of one community can be quite different from another. It falls on the public mental health director to identify the unique needs of the residents of their state as varied as they may be and to foster collaboration between systems to build a true system of care for children, adolescents, and their families. To highlight the variation in need from state to state and the manner in which different states and agencies address their unique needs this article reviews and summarizes the experiences of child and adolescent psychiatrists working intensively within the mental health systems of three different states. This approach serves to underscore the variety of leadership opportunities and skills one uses as a child psychiatrist working with state mental health systems and the necessity of developing local solutions for local problems.

MARYLAND: THE CHILD AND ADOLESCENT PSYCHIATRIST AS DIRECTOR OF STATE SERVICES

The Director of the Office of Child and Adolescent Services for the State of Maryland Mental Hygiene Administration (MHA) is a child and adolescent psychiatrist. Although not unique to Maryland, the education, skills, and understanding of the individual needs of any child that a child psychiatrist brings to such a position allows that individual to effectively advocate for a wide variety of mental health needs of children and adolescents. The following are descriptions of programs developed in the children's mental health system in Maryland that involved the child psychiatrist as director with the support and work of many others interested in children's mental health in Maryland including families, youth, advocates, other state and local agencies and academic institutions. Critical to the work in developing and expanding Maryland's system of care for children with mental health needs the director has worked with state departments including the Maryland State Department of Education (MSDE); Departments of Human Resources (DHR) (child welfare), Juvenile Services (DJS) (juvenile justice), and Disabilities; and the Department of Health and Mental Hygiene including the Mental Hygiene, Developmental Disabilities, Alcohol and Drug Abuse, Community Public Health Administrations, and Office of Maternal and Child Health and their local agency counterparts. Within the office of the director a blueprint for children's mental health was developed and is regularly updated with input from these children's mental health stakeholders from around the state. The blueprint structure guides the growth of the child and adolescent mental health system of care with subcommittees working on the major child mental health initiatives in the state.

Given the importance of early identification, assessment, and intervention, the system of care for young children ages birth to 5 years has grown over the last several years.[1,2] One indication of the need are data showing a greater number of expulsions from preschool programs than kindergarten through twelfth grade.[3] Maryland embarked on its efforts to reach young children with mental health needs early by forming an early childhood mental health steering committee co-chaired by the MHA children's mental health director and MSDE assistant superintendent for special education and early intervention. Pilot studies bringing early childhood mental health consultation[4] to child care centers in two Maryland jurisdictions were evaluated by Georgetown University and found to effectively reduce disrupted child care placements and to improve a child's growth and development. These outcomes were reported to the Governor and legislature, which led to funding to expand this consultation to all child care centers statewide. This model project underscores a common pathway for program development: research identifies a need, programs are developed, and outcome studies are then used to secure funding to expand effective programs.

Another piece of the early childhood system of care development has been early childhood mental health workforce development. Two aspects have been implemented. In collaboration with the University of Maryland child psychiatry department a certificate program was developed to train masters and above mental health professionals in early childhood mental health skills. Additionally, Maryland was chosen to implement the Center for Social Emotional Foundations of Early Learning[5] training, which promotes the social and emotional development of young children for all early childhood professionals. Trainers have been taught to use Center for Social Emotional Foundations of Early Learning because they provide training for early childhood professionals. Center for Social Emotional Foundations of Early Learning will be incorporated into a University of Maryland certificate program in the future.

Another critical area of work has been expanding mental health care in the child welfare system. Children in foster care are at high risk for mental health difficulties.[6] To prevent multiple foster care placements MHA and DHR have supported an expansion of local mental health crisis and stabilization programs with an emphasis on stabilizing foster care youth in their first foster care placement. Funding from a federal Substance Abuse and Mental Health Services Administration grant is being used to grow the use of care management entities working through a child and family team model to deliver wraparound home- and community-based services to divert foster care youth from group home and other out-of-home settings and maintain foster care youth in home- and community-based settings. A special health and mental health unit was developed for Baltimore City, which has the highest rate of youth in foster care for the state. The mental health clinicians in this unit assess all youth entering the foster care system for mental health need, participate in child and family teams, and track the follow-through of those mental health services. Programs such as this develop through the use of blending state and federal funds to address children at extremely high risk.

Youth involved with the juvenile justice system have a high level of mental health needs.[7] Collaboration continues with juvenile justice with psychiatrists and other mental health clinicians placed in all DJS detention centers to screen, assess, perform short-term treatment, and develop aftercare plans for youth entering detention. This gives an opportunity to identify unmet mental health needs. Mental health aftercare teams include mental health clinicians to ensure appropriate mental health follow-up as youth return to their community. MHA's child mental health director participates on the DJS State Advisory Board to help oversee the clinical care of youth in DJS.

Much work is done collaboratively with MSDE and local school systems. MSDE supports the use of Positive Behavior and Supports,[8] a program in individual schools throughout Maryland that fosters a supportive environment for teachers, staff, and students built on respect for others. It helps identify young people who may have mental health needs. For those students needing formal mental health assessment and treatment, school mental health programs are promoted to bring mental health clinicians to work directly in schools, bringing services that complement those provided by school staff. School health centers with mental health services are also available in many schools to provide care in communities where community health services may be more difficult to access. Students with individual education plans for mental health reasons often have some of the poorest outcomes in school. A plan to improve these outcomes is being developed with MSDE and other stakeholders.

Transition-age youth require special services because they transition from child to adult systems of care.[9] Support for independent living with job or education supports is desired by youth rather than traditional mental health services. A long-range plan to improve care for transition-aged youth has been developed, which includes standards for transition-age youth programs to help improve the consistency and quality of services.

Children's mental health workforce development is critical. A workforce committee chaired by the MHA children's mental health director and MSDE assistant superintendent for special education is looking at recruitment, retention, and training opportunities. Core competencies for workers in children's mental health have been developed with training modules for use by universities and other training entitles in the state to provide a baseline of competencies for the child mental health workforce. Information and programs to attract high school youth to careers in children's mental health have been initiated in parts of the state.

Evidenced-based practice implementation is an important area of quality service delivery for Maryland. A Child and Adolescent Mental Health Institute was formed to research, evaluate, and implement evidenced-based practices for children's mental health. A unique partnership of the child psychiatry divisions of the University of Maryland and Johns Hopkins Universities joined by the Maryland Coalition of Families for Children's Mental Health and MHA form the Institute. Implementation of trauma-informed cognitive behavior therapy, treatment foster care, wraparound service delivery, and psychopharmacology review for youth in DHR and DJS are some of the projects the Institute is involved in with other partners.

Family leadership development has been very important. Formation of the Maryland Coalition of Families for Children's Mental Health[10] has given rise to an expansion of family-to-family support services and leadership development around the state. Families participate fully in all children's mental health policy development in Maryland.

Youth leadership is equally important. Maryland has the first statewide Youth MOVE (*M*otivating *O*thers through *V*oices of *E*xperience),[11] a national youth leadership effort supporting the involvement of youth with mental health needs in policy decisions and outcome oversight.

Growing a full continuum of services to scale in all Maryland jurisdictions continues to be an important goal for MHA, families, and youth and other advocates, stakeholders, and state and local agencies in Maryland. Medicaid mental health services are developed and overseen by MHA in a fee-for-service system using an administrative services organization to perform utilization review, provider enrollment, data management, and fee payment. All levels of care are available from inpatient hospital for emergencies and short-term assessments; residential treatment centers for longer-term care; partial hospital programs; mobile treatment and in-home crisis stabilization programs; psychiatric rehabilitation programs, which include afterschool programs, skill development groups, and mentoring; one-on-one therapeutic behavioral aides; and intensive outpatient and traditional outpatient services including individual, family, and group psychotherapies. Maryland is a recipient of a Psychiatric Residential Treatment Facility 1915C Medicaid Demonstration Waiver.[12] This waiver is being used to return and divert youth who meet medical necessity criteria for residential treatment center admission. This waiver allows Medicaid funding for other important home- and community-based services not otherwise covered by Medicaid including respite care; family peer-to-peer services; youth peer-to-peer services; family education; expressive therapies (art, music, dance, equine-assisted therapies); and an in-home stabilization service. The waiver allows coverage for youth who are community Medicaid eligible and youth who were only eligible for Medicaid while in institutional care in the residential treatment centers. Care management entities manage the care of youth in the waiver using child and family teams to develop a care plan and a wraparound service delivery model to deliver services.[13] This concept of a care management entity with child and family teams and wraparound service delivery is used to expand home- and community-based services. Pilots by DHR and DJS using this model divert youth from group home and above out-of-home settings to stabilize them in home- and community-based settings. The model is also being used in the Substance Abuse and Mental Health Services Administration grant to divert foster care youth from group home settings.

Working as a child and adolescent psychiatrist in a state system is an interesting, challenging, and extremely rewarding experience. Often in treating an individual child and family in practice, the problems with child serving systems can become very apparent. Problems of collaboration between systems, lack of a full array of services, missing earlier signs of need in a child, with systems intervening too late in a child's life all can cause frustration to the treating psychiatrist. Working as a state administrator can enable one to begin to change systems and improve on these problems, potentially improving the lives of many children and families. Patience is required because true sustainable change takes many years. As the work of change proceeds, collaborating with colleagues in an array of child-serving systems helps one be patient and is a reward in itself. When change does occur, when one hears how a new program has helped one child and family, the sense of accomplishment and satisfaction in a job well done is immeasurable.

ILLINOIS: THE ACADEMIC CHILD PSYCHIATRIST AS A CONSULTANT TO A STATE CHILD WELFARE AGENCY

There are several models guiding the work of child psychiatrists in the foster care system. In one model, the Illinois Department of Children and Family Services

(DCFS), the state child welfare agency, contracts with a university-based academic child and adolescent psychiatry program (University of Illinois at Chicago division of child and adolescent psychiatry) for clinical guidance and program development.

In this model the academic child and adolescent psychiatrist, instead of working directly for the state, brings his or her expertise and the resources of a fully developed university-based department of child and adolescent psychiatry to a state agency as consultant and subcontractor. Child welfare agencies may realize extra value in partnering with academic child psychiatry programs to design and implement mental health programs for youth in foster care. Academic child psychiatry programs often carry a level of credibility not shared by clinicians in private and community settings. Additionally, academic child psychiatrists may be more familiar with and more likely to use evidence-based practices and are more likely to have access to resources and expertise necessary to design and maintain computerized databases to support the work, analyze large data sets, and design effective quality improvement programs. Finally, depending on the nature of the collaboration, the state agency may be eligible for federally matching Title IV-E money.[14] State universities are eligible for a higher rate of matching than private universities or community agencies.

Foster children (by definition eligible for Medicaid benefits) are at higher risk for developing emotional and behavioral disturbances and mental illness, use mental health services at higher rates, and are more likely to receive psychotropic medications than other Medicaid-eligible youth.[15–20] Foster children with severe emotional and behavioral disturbances present a daunting clinical challenge both to the care providers and the child welfare system as a whole. Child psychiatrists are in a unique position to provide administrative and clinical leadership to child welfare agencies. Their training provides them with an understanding of the contributions of biologic, psychologic, and social forces and the role of abuse, neglect, and trauma on the development of psychopathology in children and adolescents. Because of their broad-based expertise, child psychiatrists have a wide range of diagnostic and treatment options at their disposal, including medication management and psychotherapeutic interventions, and with their understanding of systems of care are in a unique position to design and implement comprehensive treatment plans for children in foster care. Additionally, they are well positioned to design policies and procedures and systems of care for improving psychiatric care in the child welfare system.

The University of Illinois Behavioral Health and Welfare Program

In the late 1980s and the early 1990s the Illinois Department of Children and Family Services, the state child welfare agency, faced legal challenges, including a class action lawsuit from federal investigators, advocates for children, and the American Civil Liberties Union regarding allegations of inadequate and poor quality mental health services for youth in its custody.[21] These challenges were ultimately settled through a federal court-approved consent decree in which DCFS agreed to initiate major reforms in the state child welfare system. As part of the consent decree, the University of Illinois at Chicago's department of psychiatry was identified by both DCFS and the plaintiffs as an "independent expert" to help implement the system change efforts, and an innovative collaboration was crafted between University of Illinois at Chicago and DCFS. Since 1993, DCFS officials and University of Illinois at Chicago faculty and staff have been working together to improve clinical outcomes for foster children with psychiatric and behavioral disorders. This collaboration ultimately resulted in the formation of the Behavioral Health and Welfare Program (BHWP), which consists of four separate projects with distinct but interrelated deliverables (**Fig. 1**).

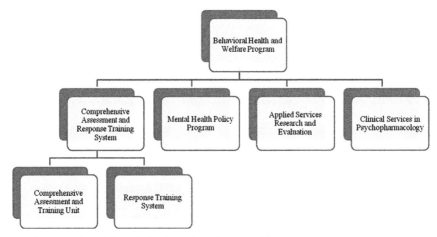

Fig. 1. Organizational chart: behavioral health and welfare program.

The Comprehensive Assessment and Response Training System

The Comprehensive Assessment and Response Training System was developed to improve the quality of psychiatric care provided to DCFS wards in residential and group home placements and to enhance placement permanence. The program consists of two components, the Comprehensive Assessment and Treatment Unit, a nine-bed psychiatric inpatient unit, and the Response Training System, a mobile consultation team that provides consultation and technical assistance to residential treatment centers and group homes.[21,22]

The Comprehensive Assessment and Treatment Unit is an acute psychiatric unit housed at the University of Illinois Medical Center at Chicago dedicated to treating the most high-end DCFS wards between the ages of 11 and 17 years. Youngsters admitted to the unit must meet criteria for an acute psychiatric hospital admission. In addition, candidates for the unit must meet two other criteria designed to screen for the most severely impaired and most difficult to manage foster children. First, the adolescent's emotional disturbance and behavioral problems have not been successfully managed in less restrictive settings, including other hospitals; have caused multiple placement disruptions; and endangers the adolescent's current placement. Typically, eligible adolescents have failed in several foster home placements, group homes, and residential treatment facilities and, by definition, have had three or more inpatient psychiatric hospitalizations in the preceding 18 months. Second, the adolescent must have a history of severe, repetitive aggression directed toward others, self, or property.

The Response Training System functions as the consultation arm of the Comprehensive Assessment and Response Training System Program. The primary goals of the Response Training System are to enhance the continuity of treatment between the hospital and the residential treatment center or group home by exporting the treatment plan to the treatment facility, to assist the residential staff in implementing discharge recommendations, to provide technical assistance to the placement, and to act as client advocates with respect to DCFS and other involved agencies.

The Mental Health Policy Program

The Mental Health Policy Program was designed to review the quality of care provided by group homes, residential treatment centers, and psychiatric hospitals serving foster children and to provide technical assistance and consultation, including training and continuing education opportunities, to community agencies that have either encountered difficulties working with high-risk populations of DCFS wards or are seeking to enhance the clinical and professional skill-set of their staff. Since its inception, the Mental Health Policy Program has conducted approximately 450 on-site reviews in Illinois and in other states where DCFS had formerly placed its wards. Services provided to community agencies include (1) an extensive program evaluation including an assessment of the treatment model, delivery of clinical services, the physical plant, and the adequacy of staffing; (2) conducting training programs for managerial staff and board of directors; (3) designing and helping implement a corrective action plan to address programmatic deficiencies identified in the program evaluation including technical assistance, consultation, and staff training aimed at helping the program develop a more effective model of care; and (4) providing consultation aimed at improving treatment planning and therapeutic outcomes with difficult client populations.

To enhance its technical assistance and consultation capacity, the Mental Health Policy Program can engage expertise from the other behavioral health and welfare programs.

Clinical Services in Psychopharmacology

Nationally, child welfare agencies have devised several mechanisms to provide consent for treatment of foster children with psychotropic medications.[23] In Illinois, the deputy director of the Office of the Guardian and Advocacy is empowered to provide consent for all youth for whom DCFS has guardianship. Guided by DCFS Rule 325,[24] the Clinical Services in Psychopharmacology (CSP) program[25] provides an independent medication review of psychotropic medication consent requests submitted by care providers for foster children. Designed to ensure the safety and appropriateness of psychotropic medication for foster children, the CSP monitors the use of psychotropic medications in this population. The CSP reviews approximately 13,000 psychotropic medication consent requests annually. In addition to reviewing medication requests, the CSP (1) provides consultation on particularly difficult or complex cases through the resources at the Institute for Juvenile Research and the Department of Psychiatry; (2) notifies the DCFS Office of the Guardian and Advocacy when local or provider patterns warrant further review and possible remediation; (3) disseminates information on new pharmaceutical developments and alerts to prescribing physicians who serve DCFS wards; (4) drafts materials and reviews and comments on DCFS-developed best practice guidelines and administrative rules and procedures governing the management of psychotropic drugs; and (5) develops training materials and conducts training for foster parents, other care providers, and DCFS-identified staff in management of psychotropic medications.

Applied Services Research and Evaluation Program

The Applied Services Research and Evaluation Program (ASREP) assists DCFS and its provider agencies in developing continuous quality improvement initiatives and data-based managerial tools for use in service monitoring, service capacity planning, and performance-based provider contracting. The ASREP works directly with DCFS and the other behavioral health and welfare programs to identify, collect, and use data concerning the problems and needs of wards with serious emotional and behavioral disorders; the mental health, placement, and social services these wards receive; and the clinical outcomes of those services.

Major Initiatives

The BHWP is currently involved in several state-wide initiatives that are transforming the delivery of   high-end mental health services to Illinois children in foster care:

1. *The Psychiatric Hospital/Residential Treatment Network.* The BHWP in conjunction with DCFS has designed a pilot project to expand the CARTS technical assistance model through the development of an innovative network of partnering psychiatric hospitals and residential treatment centers to improve the quality and continuity of care for foster children in institutional settings. The program includes a hospital-based mobile consultant that provides on-site consultation to partnering residential programs in order to export successful treatment and behavioral intervention strategies developed in the hospital to the residential treatment facility.
2. *The Illinois Residential Runaway Project.* The BHWP is spearheading an effort to decrease the frequency of elopements from residential treatment facilities and group homes and to decrease the risk a child faces while on run. Towards this end, the BHWP conducted a state-wide assessment of practices related to elopement, and collected and analyzed data relevant to running away. On the basis of these findings, guidelines were developed to help placements manage elopements more effectively.
3. *The Residential Transition and Discharge Protocol.* The BHWP in partnership with DCFS designed a protocol to promote the successful transition to a lower level of care for young people served in residential care, group homes or transitional living programs. This project involves policy changes in reimbursement to discharging and receiving placements to support the transition process and the implementation of a state-wide training program.

The opportunities for collaboration between an academic child and adolescent psychiatrist and state mental health and public welfare agencies are truly limitless. Skills as a clinician and teacher who understands child development and pathology in addition to group and system processes are highly valued within public agencies that are often struggling to address the complex needs of extremely vulnerable children and adolescents. These are often win-win situations because state agencies often can serve as sources of much needed funding for academic programs. The collaborative partnerships formed between academic child psychiatrists and state agencies are also powerful voices in advocating for the mental health needs of a state's residents.

ARIZONA: THE CHILD PSYCHIATRIST AS MEDICAL DIRECTOR OF A STATE AGENCY FOR PERSONS WITH DEVELOPMENTAL DISABILITIES

Child and adolescent psychiatrists are also well trained to provide medical leadership to agencies providing services to persons with developmental disabilities. Many factors, including their immersion in child development and systems-based practice during training, help to prepare child psychiatrists for work with both state and local agencies providing services to persons with autism, intellectual disability,[a] and other disabling conditions. Child psychiatrists may play multiple roles within these agencies, both administrative and clinical, to improve the quality of care for persons with developmental disabilities. This portion of the article describes Arizona's system of care for

---

[a] Note: This article uses the term "intellectual disability" in the place of "mental retardation."

persons with developmental disabilities and the responsibilities of the child psychiatrist–medical director within this state system.

Arizona's Division of Developmental Disabilities is one of several agencies comprising the state's Department of Economic Security. Other sister agencies include the Division of Children, Youth and Families (including Child Protective Services); the Division of Aging and Adult Services; and the Arizona Early Intervention Program. The Division provides services to over 29,000 individuals with autism, intellectual disability, epilepsy, and cerebral palsy statewide. For a number of reasons described later, the Arizona Division of Developmental Disabilities is unique among state agencies providing services to person with developmental disabilities.[26]

Arizona has one of the highest percentages of persons with developmental disabilities living in community settings and one of the smallest number of residents living in intermediate care facilities for the mentally retarded. To provide services to the large number of persons living either with their families or in group homes, the Arizona Division of Developmental Disabilities employs several hundred support coordinators (case managers) to coordinate the home-based services for the children and adolescents enrolled with the Division. This includes both long-term care and acute-care services provided by the Division as part of the State "bundled, managed care" Medicaid long-term care program. Because of the high incidence of medical problems in persons with developmental disabilities, the support coordinator's work is supported by district nurses who provide assessments in the various community settings where persons with developmental disabilities live, work, and receive services.

The child psychiatrist–medical director provides clinical support to support coordinators statewide through various means. Records may be submitted to the medical director for a clinical review and recommendations for treatment planning. The medical director may travel to provide onsite evaluations of persons with developmental disabilities and comorbid physical or mental illness. The medical director also provides training when needed on both physical and mental health issues that may affect the quality of life for individuals with developmental disabilities. Recent trainings provided by the medical director include "aging and developmental disabilities" and "choking and aspiration risk."

Arizona has only one large intermediate-care facility for the mentally retarded, which is located in Coolidge, about 70 miles south of Phoenix, housing less than 120 individuals. The Arizona Training Program at Coolidge had its admissions capped almost two decades ago, resulting in an aging population and a shift toward a more medically ill population. The Division also supports several much smaller facilities, which are primarily in Arizona's urban centers (Phoenix, Tucson, and Flagstaff). The child psychiatrist–medical director provides clinical consultation as needed to individuals residing at the Arizona Training Program at Coolidge. They also provide program oversight at the facility, providing linkage between the Arizona Training Program at Coolidge and the Division's central office in Phoenix. The medical director also attends the monthly clinical conference held with the physician providing medical care to the Arizona Training Program at Coolidge residents.

The Arizona Division of Developmental Disabilities is also unique among state programs for the developmentally disabled in that they manage their own Medicaid program for acute- and long-term medical care for its enrolled members, Arizona Long Term Care System (DD-ALTCS), under contract with the Arizona Health Care Cost Containment System (AHCCCS). The Division's support coordinators work with individuals, their families, and appointed legal guardians to provide them access to long-term care services, such as respite care, attendant care, and habilitative therapies including speech, occupational, and physical therapy (in Arizona, habilitative therapy is defined as that which is intended to assist the individual maintain a current level of functioning, in contrast with rehabilitative therapy, which is intended to help an individual return to a previously attained level of function).

The child psychiatrist–medical director provides many functions related to the administration of the DD-ALTCS program. They consult regularly with the program's administrator on both clinical and policy issues. They represent the Division in meetings with the state Medicaid agency on a variety of issues ranging from concerns about an individual's care to policy issues that affect the care of all enrolled in the program. The medical director reviews the medical records and authorizes all sterilization procedures and referrals to hospice for persons enrolled in DD-ALTCS, to ensure that the rights of persons with developmental disabilities are respected. They also review and sign off on the purchase of all durable medical equipment costing over $1000, to make certain that all purchases are medically necessary. They review and sign off on all denials and reductions in therapy prescribed by physicians for individuals enrolled with the DD-ALTCS plan, again to ensure that all ongoing therapy remains medically necessary.

The Division also manages a home modification program that assists families that are caring for their disabled family members at home. The program provides such medically necessary home modifications as wheelchair ramps, roll-in showers, and the widening of doorways to allow a wheelchair to pass through more easily. The medical director also signs off on all home modification plans to ensure the medical necessity of each request.

In addition to the long-term care services, the Division also contracts with four health plans to provide acute care services for its members. As part of its request for proposal process, the Division has strived to provide families across the state with two health plans from which to choose. The contracted health plans provide all necessary inpatient, outpatient, pharmacy, and rehabilitative therapy services. The Division's Health Care Services Unit manages the contracts with the health plans and provides oversight of the services provided, as required by the Division's contract with AHCCCS.

The child psychiatrist–medical director has learned that effective management of the Division's contracts with its health plans is based on good working relationships with each of the plan's chief medical officers. This includes being available to the health plan medical directors whenever needed to assist in management of complex medical and administrative issues and to answer questions regarding Division policy and procedure. The medical director chairs a quarterly meeting for the contracted health plan chief medical officers to obtain their input on the policies in development and in meeting the monitoring requirements of the state Medicaid agency. The medical director is also involved in the annual operational and financial review of each contracted health plan.

As part of their contract with the AHCCCS, the Division maintains a grievance and appeal process, managed by the Office of Compliance and Review. The Office manages all grievances (typically filed for denials of eligibility for state services); appeals (filed when requested services or durable medical equipment is denied); or claim disputes (when the Division denies payment for a claim filed by a contracted health plan). Those grievances and appeals that are not resolved are adjudicated at hearing in front of an administrative law judge.

The medical director is actively involved in the grievance and appeal process. They review all grievances and appeals, either upholding the denial or resolving the matter by overturning the previous decision. They also assist in the resolution of claim disputes as needed. They work with the assistant attorney general assigned to the Division before the hearing and appear in court as the Division's expert witness.

The Arizona Division of Developmental Disabilities is also unique in that it manages the behavioral health component as part of the bundled, managed care program for the delivery of all needed behavioral health services for its enrolled members. The Division contracts with the Arizona Division of Behavioral Health Services to provide these services to its members through its system of regional behavioral health authorities. Each regional behavioral health authority, in turn, contracts with several local mental health agencies to provide direct services to Medicaid-eligible individuals (including those enrolled with the Division of Developmental Disabilities). The Division's Behavioral Health Unit monitors the quality of mental health services delivered to its members by the regional behavioral health authorities and their contracted agencies.

The child psychiatrist–medical director assists the division's behavioral health manager and staff in oversight of the mental health care provided to the DD-ALTCS enrolled members by reviewing records and making recommendations for treatment and assisting in crisis resolution. They attend monthly meetings with the division of behavioral health services medical director and the regional behavioral health authority medical directors to ensure that access to all needed behavioral health services is maintained and where services are not available, to ensure that they are developed. Good working relationships with other high-level medical administrators are essential and are based on a mutual desire to provide high-quality services to all dually enrolled individuals. The medical director also helps develop Division policies regarding behavioral health services for its members and is also involved in the monitoring process to ensure that these policies are carried out by the regional behavioral health authorities.

The Division has an active quality management program that provides the required oversight of all services paid for through DD-ALTCS. The program's monitors provide both paper and on-site review of services provided by the agencies that contract with the Division to provide both child and adult foster care settings and adult group living homes, typically with two to four persons per home. The monitors also investigate care concerns brought to the attention of the Division by individuals enrolled with the Division, their guardians, or monitors at the AHCCCS. The quality management administrator oversees all aspects of the quality management program and takes the lead in the Division's preparations for the yearly operational and financial review with AHCCCS.

The child psychiatrist–medical director works closely with the quality management administrator to ensure that the Division's quality management plan is fully implemented, all needed monitoring is completed, and all needed data are collected. The medical director is also chair of the Division's statewide quality management committee, which is composed of Division employees from across the state plus selected individuals representing the Division's contracted provider agencies. The statewide quality management committee reviews the data collected by the quality management program and provides input into the Division's executive team. The medical director also reviews and signs all response letters from the Division to care concerns put forward by AHCCCS.

The medical director is also chair of the Division's mortality review committee and writes the annual mortality report. They review the initial reports on all deaths of persons enrolled with the Division and decide which of these require further review. Once the additional records have been obtained, the medical director completes a second and final review and decides which of the cases should be studied in depth by the mortality review committee. They identify those cases that represent issues of state-wide importance or those that, on further study, may result in new Division policies or changes to existing policies. The results of the medical director's case review and the mortality review committee's discussions are presented to the statewide quality management committee and to the Division's management team when policy changes are recommended.

The Division of Developmental Disability's mortality review process compares favorably with the basic components for mortality reviews conducted by agencies serving persons with developmental disabilities as identified in their May 2008 report, "Medicaid Home and Community Waivers: CMS Should Encourage States to Conduct Mortality Review for Individuals with Developmental Disabilities."[27]

The child and adolescent psychiatrist working as a medical director within a state agency has to be prepared for change, because job roles and responsibilities frequently can shift. Changes in the Governor's office, in the leadership of the Division, and in the state economy have an impact on the agency and the position as medical director. For example, within Arizona the Division of Developmental Disabilities has changed over the years from being primarily a social service agency to being both a provider of services and a health plan for its clients.

As has been the case for many psychiatric administrators,[28] this has resulted in a great deal of on-the-job self-training. Throughout this process, an understanding of system-based practice has been crucial. Remaining active with clinical work has also been quite helpful for staying in touch with the basic needs of patients and their families and for keeping one's clinical skills sharp. The rewards of serving as a state medical director have been innumerable, but collaborating and serving with clinicians and patients across the entire state has been one of the greatest.

REFERENCES

1. Knitzer J. Building services and systems to support the healthy emotional development of young children: an action guide for policymakers. New York (NY): National Center for Children in Poverty, Columbia University Mailman School of Public Health; 2002.
2. Johnson K, Knitzer J. Spending smarter: a funding guide for policymakers and advocates to promote social and emotional health and school readiness. New York (NY): National Center for Children in Poverty, Columbia University Mailman School of Public Health; 2005.
3. Gilliam WS. Prekindergarteners left behind: expulsion rates in state prekindergarten systems. New Haven (CT): Yale University Child Study Center; 2005.
4. Hepburn K, Kaufman R, Perry D, et al. Early childhood mental health consultation an evaluation tool kit. Washington, DC: National Technical Assistance Center for Children's Mental Health, Georgetown University Center for Child and Human Development; 2007.
5. Csefel. Center on social and emotional foundations for early learning. Available at: http://www.vanderbilt.edu/csefel.
6. Pires S, Lazear K, Conlan L. A primer for child welfare. Washington, DC: National Technical Assistance Center for Children's Mental Health, Georgetown University Center for Child and Human Development; 2008.
7. National Center for Mental Health and Juvenile Justice. Available at: http://www.ncmhjj.com/.
8. School-wide positive behavior support implementers' blueprint and self-assessment, Office of Special Education Programs Center on positive behavioral interventions and supports, University of Oregon. Available at: http://www.pbis.org 2004.

9. Clark HB, Davis M. Transition to adulthood: a resource for assisting young people with emotional or behavioral difficulties. Baltimore (MD): Paul H. Brookes, JS Publishing; 2000.

10. Maryland Coalition of Families for Children's Mental Health. Available at: http://www.mdcoalition.org/.

11. Youth M.O.V.E. Available at: http://youthmove.us/.

12. Centers for Medicare and Medicaid Services. Available at: http://www.cms.hhs.gov/DeficitReductionAct/20_PRTF.asp/.

13. Bruns EJ. WalkerJS. Adams J, et al. National Wraparound Initiative Advisory Group. Ten principles of the wraparound process. Portland, Oregon: National Wraparound Initiative, Research and Training Center on Family Support and Children's Mental Health, Portland State university. Available at: http://rtc.pdx.edu/PDF/TenPrincWAProcess.pdf;2004

14. US Department of Health and Human Services. Code of federal regulations, Title 45, Chapter XIII, Part 1356, Section 60,1998.

15. Burns BJ, Phillips SD, Wagner HR, et al. Mental health need and access to mental health services by youths involved with child welfare: a national survey. J Am Acad Child Adolesc Psychiatry 2004;43:960–70.

16. Halfon N, Berkowitz G, Klee L. Mental health service utilization by children in foster care in California. Pediatrics 1992;89:1238–44.

17. Harman JS, Childs GE, Kelleher KJ. Mental health utilization and expenditures by children in foster care. Arch Pediatr Adolesc Med 2000;154:1114–7.

18. McIntyre A, Keesler TY. Psychological disorders among foster children. J Clin Child Psychol 1986;15:297–303.

19. Raghavan R, Zima BT, Anderson RM, et al. Psychotropic medication use in a national probability sample of children in the child welfare system. J Child Adolesc Psychopharmacol 2005;15:97–106.

20. Trupin EW, Tarico VS, Low BP, et al. Children on child protective service caseloads: prevalence and nature of serious emotional disturbance. Child Abuse Negl 1993;17:345–55.

21. Mezey SG. Systemic reform litigation and child welfare policy: the case of Illinois. Law and Policy 1998;20:203–30.

22. Naylor MW, Anderson TR, Morris A. Child psychiatry and child welfare: a collaboration for change. Residential Treatment for Children and Youth 2003;21:33–50.

23. Naylor MW, Davidson CV, Ortega-Piron DJ, et al. Psychotropic medication management for youth in state care: consent, oversight, and policy considerations. Child Welfare 2007;86:175–92.

24. Department of Children and Family Services. Rule 325. Administration of psychotropic medications to children for whom DCFS is legally responsible. Available at: http://www.state.il.us/dcfs/docs/325.pdf. 1995.

25. University of Illinois at Chicago Clinical Services in Psychopharmacology. Available at: http://www.psych.uic.edu/cps. 2008.

26. Arizona Division of Developmental Disabilities, Department of Economic Security. 2008. Navigating the system. Available at: https://egov.azdes.gov/CMS400Min/InternetFiles/Pamphlets/pdf/DDD-1260AHBPPD.pdf. Accessed March 29, 2009.

27. Government Accountability Office. 2008. Report to the Ranking Member, Committee on Finance, U.S. Senate, Medicaid Home and Community-Based Waivers. CMS should encourage states to conduct mortality reviews for individuals with developmental disabilities (GAO-08-529). Available at: http://www.gao.gov/new.items/d08529.pdf. Accessed March 10, 2009.

28. Faulkner L. Development as a psychiatric administrator. In: Kay J, Siberman E, Pessar L, editors. Handbook of psychiatric education and faculty development. Washington, DC: American Psychiatric Press; 1999. p. 559.

FURTHER READINGS

AACAP. Practice parameters for the assessment and treatment of children, adolescents and adults with autism and other developmental disorders. Available at: http://www.aacap.org/galleries/PracticeParamters/Autism.pdf. 1999. Accessed March 27, 2009.

AACAP. Practice parameters for the assessment and treatment of children, adolescents and adults with mental retardation and comorbid mental disorders. Available at: http://www.aacap.org/galleries/PracticeParamters/Mr.pdf. 1999. Accessed March 27, 2009.

The History of Managed Care and the Role of the Child and Adolescent Psychiatrist

Martin Glasser, MD

KEYWORDS

- Children • Psychiatry • Health insurance
- Managed care • Career

The role of a physician, psychiatrist, or child psychiatrist working for a managed health care plan includes basic commitments to our profession and to ourselves. Many factors, including the Hippocratic oath, our commitment to the ethics of medical practice, our specialty and licensing requirements, federal guidelines, and our malpractice insurance carriers, all influence how we conduct our professional life. While none of our core commitments change when we accept a position to work for an organized system of care, such as a managed care organization, we acquire an additional set of expectations within that system. The purpose of this article, then, is to offer a brief history of the role that physicians have played in the development of managed care, focusing especially on the current positions that psychiatrists and child psychiatrists currently have in the system of care that we call a *managed care organization*. *Physician* in this article will mean both a psychiatrist and child and adolescent psychiatrist unless specifically stated.

It is estimated that up to 70% of practicing psychiatrists currently participate in some form of work for a managed care organization.[1] This participation can take place in many ways: contracting with a network, working as a consultant on clinical practice guidelines, reviewing quality management programs, or functioning as a paid peer reviewer to conduct utilization reviews or to demonstrate an innovative project for improving care for children and families.

Disclosures: Dr Glasser has worked for several national health plans and as a surveyor for the National Committee for Quality Assurance. He has held faculty appointments in pediatrics and psychiatry at the University of California, San Francisco as an associate clinical professor of psychiatry and pediatrics and is on the Clinical Teaching Faculty at the University of California, San Diego, Department of Psychiatry.
Behavioral Health, Anthem Blue Cross National Accounts, 9655 Gromite Ridge Drive San Diego, CA 921232658, USA
E-mail address: martin.glasser@wellpoint.com

Child Adolesc Psychiatric Clin N Am 19 (2010) 63–74
doi:10.1016/j.chc.2009.08.009   **childpsych.theclinics.com**
1056-4993/09/$ – see front matter © 2010 Elsevier Inc. All rights reserved.

Health care delivery has been in a state of change for the last 40 years, with the roles and functions of physicians changing and with new systems of care continuing to need psychiatrists and child psychiatrists in the projected systems of the future. What follows is a discussion of the history of managed care that focuses on both past and current positions as they have developed over time to meet the needs of this system of care.

HISTORY OF PHYSICIANS IN AN ORGANIZED SYSTEM OF CARE

The role of the physician paid by a system of care began within a military context: The Roman army had physicians who accompanied them into battle. Scientific evidence demonstrates that their instruments were relatively sophisticated and that their scientific accomplishments included the removal of subdural hematomas.[2] History reveals that we lost some of the knowledge of the Romans, but gradually regained the sophisticated methods of medical and surgical skills they used in combat. The United States Marine Corps brought physicians into their combat in the Spanish-American War,[3] and the practice of physicians accompanying soldiers into combat zones continues today. In 1798, the US Merchant Marine Hospital Service provided health care services for American seamen using a prepayment arrangement: Money was paid into a fund that enabled seamen to receive care for life based upon their contributions.[4]

The Veterans Administration was established in the United States in 1778. The Veterans Administration expanded the concept of a prepaid plan to include all combat veterans who were indigent or had any medical or surgical disability connected with their service.[5] This model of prepaid insurance caused organized medicine, led by the American Medical Association (AMA), to call physicians working for a salary at a government agency practitioners of "socialized medicine."[2]

This idea of prepaid insurance plans was not new. In 1945, Henry J. Kaiser and his partner Sidney R. Garfield expanded the concept of a prepaid managed care health plan to civilians. They formed an Oakland-based integrated managed care organization as a consortium of three distinct groups: the regional operating organization, Kaiser Foundation Hospitals, and the Permanente Medical Groups. Physicians hired directly by the managed care organization became part of the Permanente Medical Group to support the Kaiser Health plan and hospitals. The Kaiser Health Plans demonstrated the efficacy of exchanging health care prepayment dollars to buy a plan that paid and provided all care under a prepaid benefit. The concept of prepayment that would cover all possible health costs was one of the earliest models of the health maintenance organizations of today. By 2006, the Kaiser program employed over 12,800 physicians.[6]

Strongly protesting against any form of "lay control" over medical professionals, the AMA during the 1930s and 1940s attempted to suppress the growth of prepaid plans and cooperatives, whether they originated from the government, unions, or in any other way. The AMA expelled physicians who ran or participated in this "new delivery of health care" from their local medical societies, kept them from receiving consultations or referrals with many hospitals, and persuaded hospitals to deny these physicians admitting privileges. The behavior of the AMA resulted in their conviction in 1947 for violating the Sherman Antitrust Act. In 1950, the AMA "changed its position from official sponsorship of reprisals against prepaid group practice to watchful coexistence."[7] The AMA dropped its longstanding ban against prepaid group medical plans in 1960.[2]

CHANGES IN THE DELIVERY OF HEALTH CARE

By 1971, American medicine faced a major dilemma. The percentage of the gross national product for health care was increasing, with the majority of insured people using an indemnity health care product. Indemnity health plans followed a model that allowed a member to access any physician, who would then bill the insurance company and be paid according to a predetermined relative value scale. The member was responsible for a predetermined portion of the payment, with the majority of the reimbursement paid directly to the hospital or practitioner. The indemnity coverage did not have much oversight in regard to the use of services. The coverage or benefit still had some exclusion, such as cosmetic surgery, but the majority of all health costs were covered under the medical and behavioral health benefits.

Several covered areas in indemnity insurance were identified as high cost. These included radiology, obstetrics/gynecology, behavioral health, pharmacy, and vision. Extended inpatient and residential psychiatric care were identified as examples of high-volume and high cost usage areas with poor use management. The length of stay for youth and adults entering the inpatient psychiatric level of care often exceeded several weeks, with the length of stay for residential care for youth as long as 1 to 2 years. For-profit companies that specialized in these products owned many of the inpatient and residential programs.

In 1973, President Richard Nixon signed the Health Maintenance Organizations Act (HMO Act), a measure to address the problem of quickly escalating health care costs.[2] The stated purpose of this act was to develop new programs to encourage preventive medicine that would result in physicians engaging in and providing health care to keep people well. A primary purpose of the act was to improve the quality of health care while decreasing its cost, while at the same time also removing legal and financial barriers to the establishment of a new system of health care delivery, the health maintenance organization (HMO). Nixon offered planning grants and loan guarantees to HMOs, and authorized $375 million in federal funds to help develop HMOs and reverse some of the state regulations considered impediments to the development of HMOs. An unstated goal of the HMO Act was to reduce the cost of delivery of all health care covered by insurance and to make health care more affordable.[8] These actions resulted in the number of HMOs increasing from 30 in 1970 to 1700 in 1976. By 1980, 40 million people were enrolled in some type of a managed health care program.[2]

The Civilian Health and Medical Program of the Uniformed Services (CHAMPUS), health insurance for the dependents and retirees from the military, had an indemnity health product that was robust in its coverage and benefits. In 1987, the cost of mental health care was among this program's highest expenditure. CHAMPUS announced that they were facing insolvency due to the high cost of pharmacy, mental health, and a few other programs. To contain the costs of the CHAMPUS program, the government used an approach similar to the one used in crafting the HMO act. A pilot program, the CHAMPUS Reform Initiative, was begun in California and Virginia to determine if this model of managing the benefit could reduce the growing costs of providing mental health services to those eligible for CHAMPUS. At the same time, Congress increased the copay for psychiatric services. The CHAMPUS Reform Initiative created a restricted network of practitioners and providers whose mission was to deliver all care. To participate in this network, both the practitioner and institution had to accept a discounted rate. Also spelled out was an additional cost-containment measure that stated that all medications ordered by physicians had to be listed in a restricted formulary. Higher-cost medications or nongeneric medications were not reimbursed if a generic equivalent was available; all care was clinically managed with limits to the length of stay for residential treatment; and quality parameters and medical necessity criteria were used to manage inpatient psychiatric care.

The HMO model expanded at an exponential rate with multiple variations in the model but with the stated goal of improving the quality of care. The secondary goal was to reduce the gross national product spent on health care by providing care at a reduced cost. Physicians were asked to join these plans, with offers of increased volume of patients promised if they accepted a discounted rate of reimbursement from the HMO. Physicians started contracting with HMOs and also began participating in the development of HMOs as physician-initiated and run organizations.

The stated goal of HMO managers was to reduce the use, length of stay, and subsequent cost of mental health services. Specialized companies, called *carve-outs*, immediately sprang up.[9] These companies were often not owned or run by physicians, but rather by other mental health professionals or by businesspeople who felt that they could reduce use and, hence, the cost of the delivery of mental health care to the members of HMOs.

The concept of a carve-out was to take the high-volume, high-cost, and poorly managed components of health care (pharmacy, vision, mental health, radiology) and form specialty companies that had expertise to manage the use, improve the quality, and decrease the cost of care. The proliferation of these carve-out companies caused concerns when there were no parameters for how they functioned or uniform standards for them to follow in regard to the way they denied care.[10]

Each carve-out developed a set of guidelines called *medical necessity criteria*.[11] Decisions for access to different levels of care of mental health services, length of stay, and follow-up care were made based upon these criteria. They included requirements that members use a network of contracted mental health practitioners and institutions. The copay and deductible for mental health services were increased beyond the usual and customary payments for medical and surgical services as an attempt to decrease use. Individuals singled out in this way often saw the practice as punitive, while these methods of reducing cost were considered by the HMOs as a way to reduce the overuse of mental health services.

In just over 20 years, indemnity coverage decreased from over 90% of all health care coverage in 1970 to less than 60% of those covered in 1992. By 1995, 80% of the insured population was under some form of managed care.[12] Health plans used actuaries to project the cost of this type of care to the member. Actuaries created "road maps" identifying types of encounters a patient would have and the length of each noncomplicated encounter. The actuarial firm of Milliman and Robertson (now known as Milliman) developed "unique maps for each medical and surgical encounter as a method of clarifying the anticipated course of a patient with common medical or surgical procedures."[13] The map would trace, for example, the actions involving a patient who entered the hospital with an acute appendicitis. Day 1 would be the diagnosis and surgery. The map would document each day of the recovery with the anticipated support given to the patient and the procedures conducted. Information from this map enabled the actuaries to determine the cost of a noncomplicated procedure with data projecting how often a medical surgical encounter would occur within a stated population of individuals. The actuaries used this information to predict the cost of medical surgical health care and to then break it down to the amount of the premium paid per member per month it would cost to insure a large population of individuals. The projections were further broken down into average medical encounters and complicated health problems. They were also able to project the differences in the premium of each member per month of the delivery of health care in a Medicaid population, a commercially insured population, and a geriatric population. These projections were helpful in determining the cost of care of all medical and surgical problems, but did not cover mental health and substance abuse conditions.

Actuaries attempted to use this model to project the cost of this new system of care for psychiatric services. This was difficult to accomplish with psychiatric services because psychiatric services did not have the same road maps for psychiatric conditions and level of care as had been previously published for the medical and surgical hospital encounters. So new road maps for the noncomplicated psychiatric and substance abuse diagnoses were developed. These enabled the actuaries to use a formula that would predict the cost per member per month to provide services as projected by the actuarial guide.[14] Actuaries further expanded these guidelines to include health care for a commercial population, a Medicaid population, and a Medicare population, and for health plans that were tightly managed, well managed, or loosely managed.

The publication of the Milliman and Robertson guidelines caused an immediate protest from the American Psychiatric Association. The association stated that these guidelines were arbitrary and took away the freedom of the psychiatrist to determine what was in the best interest of each patient. "Make no mistake, we are under attack by a rapacious, dishonest, destructive, greed-driven insurance/managed-care/big business combine that is in the process of decimating all health care in America, particularly … psychotherapy and psychiatric care."[15]

The proliferation of a large number of HMOs and carved-out behavioral health organizations also created a protest from the psychiatric and medical professional organizations regarding the lack of oversight or adherence to quality standards for any of these organizations.

Statements were made that "ethics and managed care was an oxymoron."[16] The American Psychiatric Association led the charge against the mental health carve-outs, initially attacking the Milliman and Robertson guidelines as not being realistic in their projected length of stay and then by attacking the medical necessity criteria used by the managed care and specialized mental health carve-out companies. Psychiatrists working for any managed care organization were also accused of working within a system of care that had no ethics.

EXTERNAL OVERSIGHT

The rapid proliferation of managed care organizations after passage of the HMO Act created concern from consumers, large business customers, practitioners, and professional organizations that quality was not being addressed. There were concerns that physicians participating in HMOs were "gagged" from presenting the more recent clinical parameters and medications if the HMO did not offer it. Accusations were made that some HMOs offered financial incentives to the physicians in the network and to physician reviewers of use to decrease use and referrals to specialists. These concerns contributed to the formation of agencies that offered accreditation to managed care organizations and to the mental health specialty companies or carve-outs or managed behavioral care organizations.[17]

ACCREDITATION AGENCIES

In the 1990s, quality oversight of the delivery of managed care began with National Committee for Quality Assurance (NCQA) accreditation of health plans. NCQA was formed as a nonprofit company:

The National Committee for Quality Assurance is a private, 501(c)³ not-for-profit organization dedicated to improving health care quality. Since its founding in

1990, NCQA has been a central figure in driving improvement throughout the health care system, helping to elevate the issue of health care quality to the top of the national agenda.[17]

The original board of NCQA consisted of representation from unions, corporations, member advocates, and health plans. The goals were to improve the quality of care delivered to HMO members. Two methods were launched: the Health Care Effectiveness Data and Information Set performance measures and HMO standards. The Health Care Effectiveness Data and Information Set performance measures were "probes" into the total delivery system of HMOs in an attempt to measure performance and to give the public and buyers a comparison of performance. Simply stated, probes were the collection of information regarding such health measures as immunization for children, Pap smears for women, and prevention measures, such as mammograms and other accepted screening measures, collected and published as an indirect manner of determining the quality and depth of a managed care organization. The other survey tool consisted of standards measured by onsite surveys. The standards were published and given to the managed health plan prior to the survey. The standards were divided into categories under the headings Quality Management and Improvement, Utilization Management Structure, Credentialing and Recredentialing, and Enrollees' Rights and Responsibilities. The health plan was required to submit in writing a response to each standard. An onsite review was also conducted to review the documents and to conduct a randomized review of medical records for verification of proper credentialing, use review, denial procedures, and appeals procedures.[17]

As the delivery of care improved and standards were met by HMO's, the original standard would be retired with a new one replacing it. This was called "raising the bar," as a method prompting continuous improvement in the industry. The performance measures were published in a national newspaper for all readers to see which health plans provided high quality care to their members. It wasn't long before other accreditation bodies were created. Mental health services were initially not fully represented in the NCQA Managed Care Organization Standards. NCQA initiated a specialized set of standards called the Managed Behavioral Health Organization Standards in the mid-90s.

Government regulators also stepped in to develop standards to reflect a more uniform set of guidelines for mental health services. Inappropriate activities, such as "gagging" the network practitioners to prevent them from presenting noncovered or more expensive treatments, were prohibited. All medical necessity criteria that had been used by carve-outs to make use and level-of-care decisions needed to be available to the practitioners with a "due process" component to allow both the practitioner and consumer to challenge or appeal any decision made by an managed behavioral health organization. Each managed behavioral health plan applicant was also required to submit quality improvement activities. These projects were required for service and clinical activities. Each quality improvement activity submitted was reviewed for methodology, goals, and outcomes.[17]

Despite the outspoken criticism of this new system for health and mental health services, multiple advances have come out of this new system of care. NCQA has led the industry in continuously raising the threshold for higher quality care. Accreditation through the Utilization Review Accreditation Commission, the Joint Commission, and NCQA for the managed health care plans and the mental health carve-outs with additional legislation from federal and state governments continue to contribute to better health care for the members enrolled in health plans.

Over the past 10 years, consolidations have taken place among managed care organizations and managed behavioral care organizations with a decline in the number of mental health carve-outs. Managed care organizations have attracted more members. The demand for physician involvement has also increased, including demand for physicians to participate in practitioners' networks, to conduct utilization reviews with peers, and to accept employment opportunities within the health plans.

Child psychiatrists continue to be underrepresented, compared to other physicians, in managed care networks because child psychiatrists are in short supply with the demand for service in the noninsurance sector quite high. Health plans now reach out to child and adolescent psychiatrists to treat a child or adolescent by a single-case agreement with a fee negotiation. This type of agreement now brings care through private practice on a cash-only basis to the child or adolescent whose parent has a managed care policy through an employer.[18]

EMPLOYMENT IN A MANAGED CARE COMPANY

Health plans employ psychiatrists to work with health plans in several capacities. A medical director is responsible for the oversight of the program, with physician reviewers employed to use the medical necessity criteria and make decisions regarding level of care and length of stay. Psychiatrists are often employed as part-time employees.

The initial lack of uniform standards, with some gross inconsistencies among managed behavioral care organizations, has caused some physicians to consider participation in a managed care organization as similar to being a double agent, working for the "enemy" while still retaining the ethics and principles of being a physician. This concept, that a health plan is not regulated, comes from the earlier conditions of inconsistent standards and procedures and from forms of financial payment and incentives based on performance, which were removed through the influence of accreditation agencies.

While some psychiatrists remained hostile to the idea of working within a managed care system, other psychiatrists started working with the HMOs in the 1990s. Some participated on restricted panels to provide patient care reimbursed by the health plan, some worked as contracted consultants, and others were employees. The HMO movement, after 20 years, continued to generate protest from physicians, especially psychiatrists. Child and adolescent psychiatrists often remained outside of the managed care system because of the high demand for their services with no need to accept a discounted rate. All the while, the HMOs continued to recruit and use physicians and psychiatrists to support this new system of care.

A leader in management for a managed care organization was Dr Thomas Pyle. He was the medical director for the Harvard Pilgrim Health Plan, which was listed as the top health plan in the country during the time he was director. When asked about the qualifications of a physician working in a managed care organization, Dr Pyle stated:

> It is important to have people who have high ethical standards in any organization. It is important to create a culture in which people believe that costs and quality are not in opposition to one another but can work together. Systems and autonomy are not compatible—you do lose autonomy if you do what the system requires (compliance to best practices, legible entries in the medical record). It is important that everyone work within the system. A system requires ethical leaders. There must be a connection between individual ethics and the issue of systems. Physicians must go through management training. Physicians who work for a system of care must have training to connect the individual ethics and systems.[19]

Dr Pyle was clear that every physician working in a managed health care system must follow and demonstrate clear ethical standards. He added that there is also a need to demonstrate the culture of the health plan and to strictly comply with the endorsed parameters, such as the clinical practice guidelines.

PSYCHIATRISTS AS EMPLOYEES

Most Americans now have some form of a managed health plan. The psychiatrists who offer care as contracted within a network must have peer review and discussion from a psychiatrist within the health plan. Utilization for the appropriate levels of care and length of stay now follow strict guidelines for discussion with a peer, for reconsideration, and for appeals by another psychiatrist in the health plan. The roles for psychiatrists working for a health plan continue to expand. Child psychiatrists are especially in demand to assist in the development and oversight of care for children, adolescents, and families.

Managed health plans have a continuing need for child and adolescent psychiatrists to serve in networks of practitioners. The national guidelines from NCQA and other accreditation agencies state that a child and adolescent psychiatrist must be available within the managed care network within the designated time frames (emergent, urgent, or routine) or the health plan must reach out into the community and create a single-case agreement to pay for this care to be delivered. The fee may be negotiated, or full reimbursement may be paid by a one-time contract.

Other roles for physicians in a health plan include that of an advisor on a practitioner committee to reflect the standards of care in the community. The input can be in the form of a request to review the clinical practice guidelines that the health plan has adopted from such organizations as the American Academy of Child and Adolescent Psychiatry (AACAP) or the American Psychiatric Association and to modify them to reflect the standards of the local community. Reimbursements for this type of consultation are based on hourly rates. A peer must review all levels of health care. Psychiatrists conduct utilization reviews for all levels of psychiatric care. Child psychiatrist reviewers must be used when a child or adolescent psychiatrist delivers care to a child or adolescent. The peer reviewer must follow the medical necessity criteria of the health plan, but must also follow his or her personal clinical judgment concerning the best interest of the child or adolescent. National accreditation organizations, such as NCQA and the Utilization Review Accreditation Commission, prohibit any type of pressure or leverage to make a determination based upon cost or a quota.

Health plans are continuously seeking new methods of improving the quality of care to its members and to improve access to care. The integrated system of care is replacing the carve-out model of mental health care by offering an integrated model of care where mental health professionals assist pediatricians and other primary care providers to deliver care that includes mental health consultation or referral. Several innovative models of the delivery of care are funded by health plans. Descriptions of some of the models are included in this issue. Child and adolescent psychiatrists who develop, initiate, and carry out these models are often funded by a managed health plan.

Health plans must keep up to date with new medications and techniques that improve care to children and adolescents. Every major health plan has a committee to evaluate pharmacy and new technology. Child and adolescent psychiatrists also participate in these committee functions. In most health plans, the pharmacy committee includes a psychiatric medical director.

The role of a medical director working in mental health is often filled by a psychiatrist, a child psychiatrist, or an adolescent psychiatrist. This can be a part-time or a full-time role. Such a position often requires supervision and guidance to the utilization review staff and psychiatrists, but this person also reports to the executive management of the health plan.

A physician executive within such a health plan often has clinical responsibilities to the clinical staff and to the network psychiatrists. At the same time, this physician executive must also be mindful of the culture, mission statement, and values of the health plan. A physician administrator/executive actually has several roles. The job description places the physician/executive in a reporting structure that is unique to the health plan because the administrative responsibilities, clinical input, and expertise as a psychiatrist/child psychiatrist combine to make the physician executive a valuable member of a management team. The principles and ethics of the physician/executive are always primary when participating in team discussions. Dr Pyle stated that the physician leader in an executive role demonstrates high ethical values. These values are passed to the organization.

The AACAP professional Code of Ethics states: "Child and adolescent psychiatrists must not misrepresent problems, services, or diagnoses to circumvent limitations of their patient's coverage." A child and adolescent psychiatrist working for a managed care organization is always mindful of the AACAP Code of Ethics.[20]

The national accreditation agencies and the legislative governing bodies have created an atmosphere with managed mental health organizations that have made it easier to work, function, and contribute as an employee in a managed care organization, with similar medical necessity criteria, quality oversight, and regulations concerning the patient's rights and advocacy.

WHAT SHOULD YOU ASK PRIOR TO ACCEPTING A POSITION WORKING FOR A MANAGED HEALTH PLAN?

This article describes the multiple roles in which a psychiatrist can be employed by a managed care organization or a managed behavioral care organization. Prior to working with an organization, it is important to know precisely how the position that you will be accepting is defined.

If you elect to join a network of practitioners, you are required to sign a contract. The contract must state your right to share treatment modalities with your patient regardless of the covered health benefit, your ability to speak with a peer if care is denied, your ability to appeal a decision, and your financial remuneration. In addition, some contracts prohibit balance billing, the difference between what you are reimbursed and what your normal charges are for the service provided. Other contracts allow a negotiation with the patient regarding payment beyond what is reimbursed to the practitioner.

The positions of part-time or full-time employment must be completely stated in the job description for the position. A psychiatrist must always have the ability to make a clinical decision based upon ethical, fair, and honest principles. A contract that places the psychiatrist in a restricted position of signing and approving decisions made by others with no ability to use his or her clinical judgment is considered a "doc in the box" and should be avoided.

Each managed care organization has internal policies and procedures. The potential conflict raised by Dr Pyle reminds us that we must follow both the ethics and clinical parameters of the AACAP and the American Psychiatric Association, but also follow the internal procedures of the managed care organization. This is usually easy to do when the practice parameters and the level of care policies reflect the AACAP practice parameters and the level-of-care tools of the AACAP. If a managed care company does not share the nationally accepted practice parameters, acceptance of a position in this company would require the psychiatrist to use the policies and parameters accepted by the company. This is a position that can raise major ethical issues for the psychiatrist.

Prior to signing any employment contract, the culture of the managed care organization must be closely examined. This should include a review of the core values and guiding behaviors of the organization. The leading managed care organization states as core principles: the customer first, working as a team, personal accountability for excellence, and personal integrity (acting ethically, honestly, and fairly and being consistent in word and deed).[21]

Prior to employment, one should determine whether the managed care organization is accredited by NCQA, the Joint Commission, the Utilization Review Accreditation Commission, or another national accreditation agency. If accredited, the organization must follow the nationally accepted standards that each agency dictates. This ensures the ability of the psychiatrist to use best clinical practices and judgment for the member.

The delivery of health care today uses the principles of managed care for all health care products. Systems of care, Medicaid, Medicare, commercial and self-funded health plans use every possible resource to oversee the delivery of health care.

Psychiatrists are now contracted or employed in the roles defined in this article.

THE FUTURE

The model, system, and function of the delivery of psychiatric care to children and families will continue to change. This is inevitable in order to offer systems of care that can meet the needs of all individuals in our society, regardless of race or amount of money available to them. If our goal is to offer psychiatric services to children, adolescents, and families in our society, we must participate in the formation, delivery, and oversight of new systems for the delivery of this care. Our contribution can be as professionals who bring to the organization knowledge, professional ethics, and peer awareness. The challenge is for child and adolescent psychiatrists who become physician executives to be willing to learn and participate in the corporate culture of management while still adhering to their ethics and professional guidelines.

Some psychiatrists will continue to work with various systems of care employed as contracted or part-time employees. Many child psychiatrists will elect to work in an office with fee for service provided at the initiation of a session. Because of a shortage of child psychiatrists and the rising demand for services, an increasing number of child and adolescent psychiatrists over the last 10 years have decided not to participate in managed care systems of care.

Child psychiatrists have always struggled with being in demand and not needing to participate in a managed care network, and this tendency will continue as long as the demand for child psychiatrists exceeds the supply. For many of us, this creates a personal dilemma: Do we only serve children and families who can afford our fees, or do we reach out to children and families who participate in health plans that are managed?

SUMMARY

Health care is not affordable for every child and family. At any given time, there are around 50 million Americans, or 18% of the population under the age of 65, without any form of health insurance.[22] For those who are insured, the majority receives their insurance benefit as part of their employment package; employers are now seeking quality outcomes and reduction in costs. New systems for the delivery of health care are being developed to meet the needs of all Americans, wealthy or poor. These systems are being structured to resemble current managed health plans by including combinations of quality demands, utilization oversight, and access to health care professionals, while keeping plans affordable. In this way, those who provide health care will be able to create new systems of care that can engage the 18% not presently insured and to continue a full spectrum of health care for those who remain insured.

Psychiatrists can contribute to this delivery of health care by participating in the development of new systems of care, be it as employees of managed care or through contracts or other areas of participation. While there will continue to be challenges for child and adolescent psychiatrists to find a balance in appropriate reimbursement for the specialized care we deliver, we must nevertheless attempt to ensure that all children and families receive appropriate mental health services.

Child and adolescent psychiatrists have an ability to focus the system of care on the child and family. Children and adolescents are at present underserved for psychiatric problems. New initiatives request that the pediatrician and primary care physician screen adolescents for depression and screen newborns and their mothers for parent/child issues, including postpartum depression. This additional screening will create a challenge for the pediatrician to access and consult with psychiatrists for their patients who need psychiatric care. All of these factors create a greater need for an integrative model, one in which child and adolescent psychiatrists participate in a managed psychiatric system of care.

Even though the history of managed care has had its ups and downs, it now appears that many of the stumbling blocks have been worked out, bringing together the best of fee-for-service care and the original HMO template to create a system that encapsulates the best of both. In this way, more people can be served in better ways and physicians can practice medicine in ways that allow them to behave ethically. It has taken a while to get to this point, and the physician who finds himself or herself in the position of administrator needs to remain aware of the delicate balancing act of being a professional first while following the core principles and policies of the managed health plan. Such a position requires a wisdom perhaps not seen in the practice of medicine for many decades.

REFERENCES

1. Sturm R, Ringel J. The role of managed care and financing in medical practices: How does psychiatry differ from other medical fields? Soc Psychiatry Psychiatr Epidemiol 2003;38(8):427–35.
2. Managed Care Museum. Available at: http://www.managedcaremuseum.com. Accessed March 2009.
3. The National Archives. Available at: http://www.archives.gov/publications/prologue/1998/spring/spanish-american-war-marines-2.html. Accessed March 2009.
4. Marine Hospital Service. Available at: http://en.wikipedia.org/wiki/Marine_Hospital_Service. Accessed March 2009.
5. United States Department of Veterans Affairs. VA History. Available at: http://www.va.gov/about_va/vahistory.asp. Accessed March 2009.
6. History of Kaiser Permanente: about Kaiser. Available at: http://www.managedcaremuseum.com/timeline.htm.
7. Time Magazine. Medicine: AMA Indicted, January 2, 1939.
8. Managing managed care, a history of managed care. (n.d.). Retrieved from Managed Care Act of 1973. Available at: http://www.ask.com/bar?q=Managed+care+act+of+1973&page=1&qsrc=2106&ab=3&u=http://www.managingmanagedcare.com/Resources/HxMgdCare.htm.

9. Grazier KL. Effects of a mental health carve-out on use, costs, and prayers: a four-year study. J Behav Health Serv Res 2002;37(6):1583–601.

10. Busch S. Specialty health care, treatment patterns, and quality: the impact of a mental health cave-out on care for depression. Health Serv Res 2002;37: 1583–601.

11. SAMHSA'S National Mental Health Information Center. Medical necessity in private health plans. Available at: http://mentalhealth.samhsa.gov/publications/allpubs/SMA03-3790/table02.asp. Retreived March 2009.

12. BlueCross BlueShield Association. History of Blue Cross Blue Shield. Available at: March. http://www.bcbs.com/about/history/1990s.html. Accessed March 2009.

13. Our Roots. 2009. Milliman Available at:http://www.milliman.com/why-milliman/our-roots. Accessed March, 2009.

14. Glasser M. Milliman and Robertson Psychiatric ORGS.1991.

15. Eist HI. (n.d.). Volunteers in psychotherapy. Retrieved from Volunteers In Psychotherapy. Available at: http://www.ctvip.org/web2b.html.

16. Pyle T. The reformation of the health care system. The Internist 1995;36(1):13–6.

17. O'Kane M. Essentials of managed health care, accreditation and performance measurement programs for managed care organizations. Chapter 23: p521–51. Sudbury (MA): Jones and Bartlett Publishers; 2003.

18. AACAP Managed Care Pamphlet, information for parents. Washington, DC: American Academy of Child and Adolescent Psychiatry, 2008.

19. Pyles T. What's the ethics of that? A conversation with Thomas O. Pyle. Health Aff 2008;27(1):143–50.

20. AACAP Code of Ethics. Washington, DC: American Academy of Child and Adolescent Psychiatry, 2009.

21. WellPoint Core Values. Indianapolis (IN): WellPoint Health Plan Inc; 2009.

22. Alonso-Zaldivar R. USA's uninsured have yet to show collective power. Associated Press, USA Today 2009.

Overview of Practice Management in Child and Adolescent Psychiatry

Robert K. Schreter, MD

KEYWORD

• Overview of practice management

The dictionary tells us that to "administer" is to "supervise or oversee," and that to "manage" is to "direct with a degree of skill, to be in charge."[1] The administrator in child and adolescent psychiatry must create and direct a clinical delivery system, design and oversee the administrative services necessary to support the system, and guide the business operations that contribute to its success.

Psychiatric practices range in size from those of solo clinicians practicing alone in an office, to single and multispecialty group practices, to large integrated systems, both public and private. As practices expand to include a greater number of patients, clinicians, locations, services, and payers, the clinical and administrative tasks become more complex, challenging, and expensive. But regardless of the size of the practice, the psychiatrist administrator must handle seven core administrative responsibilities and oversee the individual functions and capabilities within each domain. These seven core responsibilities are practice development, clinical services management, medical office operations management, clinical care management, information management, business operations management, and risk management.

Psychiatrists, by training and temperament, are likely to demonstrate greater comfort and skill with the clinical aspects of practice than with the administrative and financial aspects. But whether the physician is an employee, independent contractor, officer of the company, partner, or owner, he or she must master practice management principles and processes. The ability to provide quality care, particularly to populations of patients, requires an administrative infrastructure and access to a comprehensive, multilevel clinical delivery system. Shepherding financial and clinical resources while earning a living demands sound financial management skills.

University of Maryland School of Medicine, Johns Hopkins School of Medicine, 2360 West Joppa Road, Suite 222, Lutherville, MD 21093, USA
E-mail address: schreters@aol.com

Child Adolesc Psychiatric Clin N Am 19 (2010) 75–87
doi:10.1016/j.chc.2009.09.001
1056-4993/09/$ – see front matter © 2010 Elsevier Inc. All rights reserved.

Clinicians are challenged to remain loyal to medicine as a calling while running their practices, organizations, and systems as a business.

This article provides an overview of the management of psychiatric practices summarized here in **Box 1**. The goal is to provide a roadmap for creating and sustaining successful clinical and administrative endeavors. The article serves as a checklist to permit beginning individuals and organizations to identify the crucial tasks and challenges. It can also be used as an audit instrument by existing practices to assess current operations so that strengths and opportunities for improvement and growth can be identified.

Box 1
Overview of practice management in child and adolescent psychiatry

Practice development

Practice model

Legal structure

Marketing

Financing

Mission, vision, values

Clinical services management

Clinical services as products

Clinical services to fill a niche

Clinical services as a function of staffing

Clinical services along the continuum of care

Innovation-driven clinical care

Medical office operations

Patient registration and scheduling

Billing and collections

Medical record keeping

Clinical and administrative policies and procedures

Cost accounting and budgeting

Personnel management

Clinical care management

Case management

Utilization management

Quality management

Outcomes management

Resource management

Information management

Internal and external communication

Technology planning

Patient confidentiality

PRACTICE DEVELOPMENT

Practice development encompasses those tasks that contribute to the creation, maintenance, and growth of the practice and that are the building blocks for practice start-up and expansion. These include those tasks related to legal, clinical, administrative, financing, accounting, and staffing issues. Practices must design formal plans to channel their efforts in the most productive directions. As a first step, individuals and colleagues must arrive at a vision of what they hope to accomplish and must create a vehicle for achieving this goal.

Traditional psychiatric services can be delivered in settings as small as a single clinician practicing independently in a sublet office and supported by only an answering machine and a computer. Some psychiatrists join colleagues in office-sharing arrangements for support and to save on overhead. In recent years, the emergence of managed care in the public and private sectors has spurred the formation of larger groups of clinicians and delivery systems capable of providing services on contractual basis to large populations of patients over wide geographic areas. To serve these contracts, clinicians have united into single and multispecialty behavioral group practices and independent practitioner organizations in which clinicians relate to each other only to provide a service to a fixed population. Larger systems include fully integrated group practices and practices embedded within larger systems, including hospitals, academic medical centers, or other integrated systems of care. Each model has benefits and drawbacks. Clinicians choose the model that best supports their expectations and plans.

Legal Structure

Most practicing clinicians and groups opt for a legal structure that insulates their personal assets from claims originating from their professional activities. Larger corporate entities look for arrangements that also permit the inclusion of partners and the ability to sign contracts with payers and providers. For larger organizations, attorneys draw up articles of incorporation, corporate bylaws, and operating agreements, which define ownership, the decision-making process, and the relationship of various participants. Participation agreements define each member's obligations and responsibilities. Compliance with state and federal regulations is crucial. For liability protection, individuals and small groups often choose such structures as limited liability corporations and S corporations. Larger organizations create more elaborate corporate structures capable of generating investment capital. Some even go public.

Marketing

Clinicians no longer receive patients exclusively from traditional referral sources. Instead, patients are now channeled through distribution arrangements that result from managed care and other contracting. This change forces clinicians, networks, and delivery systems to rethink how they maintain adequate patient volume.[2] A marketing plan is a useful way of addressing this problem. A marketing plan must include at least the following components: market analysis, payer mix, service mix, and pricing structure.[3] A market analysis is a survey of the population of potential patients surrounding your practice. The market analysis may include such information on the population of potential patients as age, socioeconomic bracket, education, location of residence, and what services they want and need. Payer mix describes the percent of your patients (and your income) that can be expected to come from self-pay, commercial insurance, managed care–reduced fee-for-service, contracts, or other revenue sources. Service mix represents the services or products you make available to the marketplace. Some services can be viewed as your "bread and butter," such as individual psychotherapy with medication management and medication management with patients in the care of nonphysician providers. Other services can be designed to create practice name identification and niches, such as forensic evaluations or the treatment of child and adult attention deficit hyperactivity disorder.

Pricing of services should be driven by community standards and your business plan. Conduct an informal survey of pricing in your community before setting your fees. Research strategies for ascertaining market rates for services must be in compliance with federal laws regulating anticompetitive behavior. Generally, one must scrupulously avoid directly exchanging price information with other health care providers offering similar services. Providers are allowed, however, to participate in surveys managed by a third party gathering information about rates and business costs. These surveys are commercially available and can be a useful source of information for providers seeking to establish market-competitive rates.[4]

Recognize that some services are reimbursed more highly than others because they are more desirable to managed care entities or other purchasers. Other services, such as marital counseling, may not be reimbursed by health insurance dollars and can be priced independently of insurance rates. Last is the development of a marketing plan that targets consumers and highlights marketing activities.[5] Individuals and small groups rely on less expensive activities, such as direct mailing, speaking, teaching, making professional presentations, conducting research, and scheduling drop-in visits. Larger organizations pay for advertising, fund marketing visits and luncheons to referral sources, sponsor special events, engage in public relations, and attend trade shows.

Formal Planning

As practices grow larger and more complex, formal planning processes return greater value. A crucial step is the creation of mission, vision, and values statements.[6] The mission statement defines the immediate purpose of the organization, identifies its customers and stakeholders, and describes the products and services it will offer. The vision statement complements the mission statement by describing what the organization hopes to achieve. An accompanying values statement articulates fundamental principles that will guide the organization's development, underpin its culture, and shape its business practices.

Financing

Capitalization is the process by which clinicians obtain money to start and grow their practices. Early in their practice, independent clinicians and small practices usually rely on personal and family savings, small bank loans, and home equity loans. They may also use a portion of their accounts receivable to fund practice growth. Larger practices and systems often partner with hospitals or other entities, borrow from the conventional marketplace, or rely on revenue from contracts for services.

CLINICAL SERVICES MANAGEMENT
Clinical Services as Products

Clinicians think of the interventions they provide as services. It is also possible to think of clinical services as products attached to revenue streams. The services offered by a clinician are usually determined by the clinician's training, skills, and interests.

Clinicians specialize by age—child, adolescent, adult, or geriatric—and by service—medication management, eclectic psychotherapy, or cognitive behavioral therapy.

Clinical Services to Fit Niches

Clinicians can also develop special services to treat special populations—attention deficit hyperactivity disorder, developmental disabilities, children from families of divorce.[7] Larger practices can expand these niche interventions to create programs, such as a multispecialty approach to the treatment of children with attention deficit hyperactivity disorder and learning disabilities, comprehensive programs to treat traumatized children, and consultation programs to schools on a contractual basis.

Clinical Services as a Function of Staffing

Larger practices can expand their services and extend their product line through staffing and hiring decisions. The addition of psychologists permits academic testing and may expand the fee range for psychotherapy. Case management can be offered by staff social workers. Nurse practitioners and physician assistants expand capacity for medication management. The inclusion of substance abuse counselors adds even another dimension—or product line—and permits an integrated approach to a dual diagnosis.

Clinical Services Along the Continuum of Care

A clinical continuum is an array of services that varies by location and extends from office-based care through community-based service to inpatient care. Another way to visualize this medical continuum is from least intensive and least restrictive services to most intensive and most restrictive services. Patients may view the clinical continuum as an array of services from which they select, mix, and match based on need, convenience, preference, and cost. Individual clinicians and small practices must be able to triage patients to appropriate levels of care along the clinical continuum. Large practices and systems can actually provide care and generate revenue at multiple levels. The following clinical care components of a delivery system provide opportunities for clinicians, practices, and systems to develop expertise and expand products[8]

- A 1-800 centralized intake system accessible 24 hours per day, 7 days per week
- Services to children, adolescents, adults, and special populations
- A wide range of outpatient services, including services to individuals, families, and groups, and medication management
- Emergency evaluation and hospital diversion
- Mobile crisis response team
- Community-based services, including wrap-around and other home-based services
- Intensive outpatient programs for psychiatric and substance abuse disorders
- Respite beds
- Evening and weekend partial hospital programs
- Twenty-three-hour inpatient and stabilization beds
- Residential treatment programs
- School-based services, including after-school programs and in-school consultation

Individuals and practices can expand their market share and increase revenues by developing innovative products. Examples may include employee assistance programs providing treatment in the workplace and school-based consultation and treatment programs providing care to children and adolescents in the educational setting. Telepsychiatry enables clinicians to extend access to care to distant locations. Community-based services need consultation and medical support. Colocating a child and adolescent psychiatrist in a pediatric practice is a win-win for patients and providers.

MEDICAL OFFICE OPERATIONS MANAGEMENT

Regardless of its size, a practice is a business whose product is the delivery within budgetary constraints of a range of health care services to individuals and populations scattered over wide geographic areas. The independent clinician must develop management competencies and devote adequate time to the task. Large groups must have competent managers on staff and commit the dollars necessary to support their administrative infrastructure. Management areas of importance to child and adolescent psychiatrists are reviewed below.

Patient Intake and Scheduling

Effective patient intake and scheduling can contribute to increased practice volume, market share, and profitability. Patients must be registered, and the necessary demographic and insurance information recorded. The practice must be sure care is authorized and that the time windows are promptly triggered. A cancellation policy must be in place and enforced. Access for emergencies must be available 24 hours a day, 7 days per week.

Billing and Collections

Billing options range from as simple as manually circling dates on a preprinted form, to using inexpensive software designed for solo practitioners and groups, to complicated software and hardware systems costing millions of dollars and designed to perform thousands of functions for the staff of a large health system. Soon, small practices as well as larger systems must be able to submit bills, including batch billing, electronically. Systems must be able to match charges with copays, third-party reimbursement, and discounts, as well as ensure authorization dates have not expired. Accounts receivable management and attention to collection rates and timeliness must be monitored.

Medical Record Keeping

Practices small and large rely on the medical record to document patient history and treatment, drive clinical decision making, inform treatment planning, and provide a defense against patient complaints of malpractice. The Institute of Medicine recently called attention to the benefits a centralized electronic medical record can contribute to patient safety.[9] Health care policy makers predict cost savings from the adoption of electronic medical records, although these savings may not be realized. Large practices and systems of care value electronic medical records because they make it possible to more quickly gain access to patient data from a distance and in emergencies. These records also make it possible to store data necessary to keep track of authorizations and alert clinicians to submit outpatient treatment reports for continued care. Other important medical data included in the medical record are *Diagnostic and Statistical Manual of Mental Disorders, Fourth Edition (DSM-IV)* diagnoses, treatment plans, short-term goals, and long-term goals, which managed care payers require for continued care. Another important function of medical records is to provide documentation of services provided to defend against billing fraud in case of an audit.

Clinical and Administrative Policies and Procedures

Compliance with Health Insurance Portability and Accountability Act (HIPAA) regulations already requires all but solo provider offices, which may not need to transmit information electronically, to show the ability to develop policies and procedures. Larger practices and corporate entities need additional policies and procedures in place. These include human resources policies to address such areas as pay, attendance, and performance. Office management policies provide job descriptions and delineate how employees are to perform their tasks. Clinical policies and procedures include treatment guidelines, medical necessity criteria, and an appeals process to respond to denial of continued care.

Cost Accounting and Budgeting

Practices must develop and implement budgets to achieve the organization's goals. Solo practices can accomplish this with paper and pencil. Large practices must have more sophisticated internal controls as well as processes of external review. The revenue cycle must be understood and monitored to enhance collections. Overhead items, such as payroll and shared purchasing, must be optimized.

Credentialing/Provider Enrollment

Clinicians must remain current with licensing entities, including state medical boards, the Drug Enforcement Administration, the issuer of the National Provider Identifier (NPI) number, hospital affiliations, public and private payers, managed care organizations, and their malpractice insurer. Larger practices routinely have a single individual responsible for ensuring that everyone in the organization has kept their credentialing current. Practices must not only make sure that the clinical staff have up-to-date credentials, but they also must manage network affiliations of all staff in accordance with the business plan for the practice.

Personnel Management

As groups get larger, the human resources function becomes more complex. Human resources is responsible for recruiting and retaining staff, contracting with employees, and monitoring provider and employee performance against benchmarks. Tasks related to administrating clinician compensation, benefits, incentives, and bonuses are all additional management functions in this area.[10] Internal training on clinical and administrative issues becomes increasingly essential as the organization becomes larger and more dispersed.

CLINICAL SERVICES MANAGEMENT

Historically, clinicians have viewed clinical management as the work of external watchdogs whose only purpose is to deny care. However, patients and payers are increasingly holding providers accountable for cost, quality, and clinical outcome. In this new environment, clinical care now extends beyond traditional treatment to include clinical management of these services.

Case Management

Clinical managers have long recognized that 20% of the patients consume 80% of the health care dollar. With an eye to reducing total cost, case managers now focusing on these high-using patients are creating individual treatment plans that best address their unique needs.[11] For example, an innovative program might allot a predetermined amount of money (eg, $50,000) to a case manager who is responsible for spending these dollars on the ideal mix of services, which could include modifications to the living situation, counseling, medications, education, after-school programming and tutoring, vocational training, in-home support services, and other wraparound services.

Use Management

Clinicians, care managers, payers, and policy makers are all concerned about how services are used. At the level of the individual patient, use is tracked through patient authorization, precertification, and the submission of outpatient treatment reports for continued care. At the system level, systems can review use of inpatient care for a population by tracking the percent of a population that require admission, frequency of readmission, and average length of stay, as well as total cost for admission. Outpatient care and costs can be evaluated by identifying the percent of a population that has actually received outpatient care, use of services by *Current Procedural Terminology* (*CPT*) code and provider, number of sessions in each episode, and the total cost of care by episode. This information is essential for contracting, budgeting, developing programs, and determining whether the right patients are being seen for the right problems at the appropriate level of care.

Quality Management

Quality management systems are designed to improve health care delivery and ensure patient safety.[12] Basic quality assurance programs are often implemented through medical record review, which compares the record against codified standards, analyzes data from patient satisfaction surveys, or monitors patient complaints. More sophisticated quality management approaches may involve continuous assessment of a set of indicators reflecting processes of care and clinical outcomes. The quality indicators may evaluate goals and objectives for the practice, such as the implementation of clinical "best practices" for the management of specific clinical syndromes. Quality improvement programs examine an area of underperformance, identify crucial deficiencies, design and implement corrective action plans, and remeasure to determine whether the interventions have actually enhanced quality. Clinicians, larger practices, and systems benefit when enhanced quality leads to improved service, enhanced outcome, and patient satisfaction, all of which contribute to enhanced practice reputation and market share.

The National Committee for Quality Assurance (NCQA) measures psychiatric quality of care by healthcare effectiveness data and information set (HEDIS) measures. One such measure is the percent of patients in the covered population who are seen in psychiatric follow-up within 30 days of discharge from a hospital to assess adequacy of follow care. A second HEDIS benchmark is the percent of a population seen for psychiatric services as a measure of the adequacy of access to services. Note that NCQA and HEDIS are designed to improve the quality of health insurance programs. Nonetheless, providers that include relevant HEDIS measures in their quality improvement plans can improve the health of populations and may be rewarded by health plans with increased referrals and pay-for-performance reimbursements.

Outcomes Management

A crucial issue for all involved in health care is whether patients benefit from the services they receive.[13,14] The demand for evidence-based medicine has intensified even as the challenges in study design, interpretation, and cost become better appreciated. But it is essential that clinical decision making for individual patients and populations be driven by data that identify which patients experience the best results in the hands of which providers of which services.

Resource Management

In fee-for-service care, clinicians are reimbursed retrospectively for the services they provide. Under managed care capitation and other at-risk contracting, provider groups are often charged with the task of providing services under global budgets. In a capitated contract, the clinician is not only responsible for the patient in front of him, but also for all other patients in the community who have not yet presented for care or will only be identified through screening and case finding. Under a capitated contract, payment is usually made on a per-member-per-month basis. The amount of the payment is calculated by multiplying the number of "covered lives" or members of a health plan eligible for the services provided by the contractually agreed upon per-member-per-month rate. The evaluation of these contract proposals requires actuarial data predicting use of services for the group of covered lives. The current drive toward health care reform can be expected to increase clinician involvement in systems that must shepherd limited resources to provide the maximum benefit for the larger society and mediate between competing claims and claimants.

INFORMATION MANAGEMENT

Management information systems make it possible to store, retrieve, use, and analyze data crucial to operating the medical office and the medical enterprise. Management information systems are relied upon to contribute a range of functions.[15]

Communication

Management information systems provide the pathways for internal communication and communication with external individuals and organizations.

Technology Planning

Anticipating information needs should be based on an assessment of the practice's services, responsibilities, relationships, and business demands. This snapshot will assist in identifying immediate hardware, software, and telecommunication needs, as well in planning for expansion.

Ensure Patient Confidentiality

Management information, such as patient registration information, account information, and claims data, should be protected similarly to clinical information. Under the force of HIPAA, it is essential for every organization to maintain an information system that protects patient and practice confidentiality and data.

Manage Clinically Relevant Material

In addition to the clinical record, management information systems will need to manage symptom checklists, screening tools, information for patients on risks and benefits, releases, and outcomes data. In addition to supporting treatment and driving clinical decision making, these data are used for authorization, use, and pay-for-performance models.

Provision of Mandated Reports

Data systems will need to track and organize data for individual reports, such as reports on outpatient treatment and cost/benefits.[16] They must also produce aggregated data, such as percent of a population's covered lives seen for clinical care during a contractual period. If pay for performance becomes an economic reality, the ability to collect, aggregate, and analyze data will be rewarded financially.

BUSINESS MANAGEMENT

Individual clinicians and large organizations clarify their mission, vision, and values early in their development. Such statements help shape the next stages of business development and management.[17] Issues in the management of these businesses are reviewed below.

Strategic Planning

The strategic plan identifies the organization's goals and describes how it intends to get there. It represents a roadmap for the future.

Business Planning

Business plans typically spell out how the organization will develop products and services and how it will make money from offering such products and services. Business plans include a marketing plan, an operations plan, a staffing plan, and also a financial plan to predict profit and loss.

Financial Planning and Oversight

The financial plan, an organizational budget, is a plan for generating income and predicting costs of necessary goods and services.[18] It also includes funding sources and an analysis of business risks and challenges. At the end of this process, it should be possible to anticipate profits and losses. Having established a budget and anticipated operating costs, financial decisions are made to reduce costs and improve revenues and profits. Regardless of the size of the clinical entity, it is important to have internal processes for managing the revenue cycle, improving collections, maintaining controls for cash management, and paying clinicians.

Maintaining Relationships with Outside Vendors

Succeeding at the business aspects of practice requires relationships with landlords, accountants, lawyers, suppliers, and other entities.

Negotiating with External Vendors and Organizations

Profitability depends on paying attention to the bottom line. Effective negotiating with vendors for goods and services, as well as clinical partners, such as hospitals, managed care organizations, and other payers, contributes to practice success.

RISK MANAGEMENT

Risk management programs are designed to increase patient safety and protect patients and providers from the consequences of untoward clinical or administrative events. Components of comprehensive risk management programs include insurance; a critical incident review process; a complaint process; processes to ensure compliance with hospital, state, and federal laws and regulations; and standing committees and manuals.

Insurance

Individual clinicians and small groups typically carry only malpractice coverage, which covers professionals for negligence by act or omission for care that deviates from community standards and results in injury or death.[19] Child and adolescent psychiatrists routinely carry this insurance in the amount of $1 million per claim and $3 million per year. Occurrence policies cover all care rendered in a policy year regardless of when the claim of negligence is made. Claims-made policies cover only claims filed during the year in which the policy is in effect. A "tail" can be purchased to extend a claims-made policy into the future for the clinician's protection. Larger entities and more complex corporate structures often need insurance coverage for their expanded activities and greater risks. These include vicarious liability coverage, errors and omissions insurance, and directors and officers insurance. Vicarious liability coverage protects "superiors" from acts of a third party for which he or she may bear right or duty to oversee or control. Errors and omissions insurance is a business protection policy that protects the business from liability for mistakes that cause financial harm to others.[20] Directors and officers insurance protects officers and the company from financial costs for damages and defense costs arising out of alleged errors, breaches in judgment of duty, or wrongful acts related to their organization's activities.[21]

Critical Incident Review

Proactive organizations have processes in place to identify critical incidents as sentinel events, which are studied to isolate systemic flaws and errors and addressed in a corrective action plan. Examples of critical incidents include inpatient admissions, suicides, patient assaults, and malpractice claims.

Complaint Process

The examination of complaints from patients, employees, and other providers offers an opportunity to improve processes and procedures.

Compliance with Hospital, State, and Federal Laws and Regulations

Practices are subject to reporting requirements from a range of overseers: insurers in the event of potential suits, social service organizations in the event of patient abuse, conflict of interest under Stark legislation. Compliance with rules regarding fraud and abuse in billing and coding must be carefully ensured. Internal auditing on a regular basis may be invaluable in this regard. Larger organizations often devote substantial resources to ensuring compliance with applicable laws and regulations.

Standing Committees and Manuals

Larger organizations have committees responsible for reviewing manuals, policies, and procedures designed to enhance safety and reduce risk. Committees routinely review critical incidents, examine complaints, oversee compliance with business and government requirements, review medical record review processes, and compare employee performance to standards.

SUMMARY

As health care costs in America continue to climb toward 16% of the capital gross domestic product, there is emerging consensus that health care reform may soon become a reality. It is impossible to predict, with certainty, what exact shape this reform will take, in what sequence different components will be enacted, and what impact it will have on psychiatric practices and delivery systems. It is likely that providers will be held increasingly accountable for quality, cost, and outcome.[22,23] During the early years of managed care in the late 1980s and early 1990s, independent clinicians and small groups were under significant pressure to merge into larger practices, networks, and systems.[24,25] History may repeat itself in this upcoming round of health care reform. If this happens, the seven areas of practice management and the individual capabilities and capacities within each domain highlighted in this article will provide clinicians with a roadmap for adapting to the transformations in health care payment and delivery.[26]

REFERENCES

1. The Merriam-Webster dictionary. New York: Simon & Schuster; 1974.
2. Davis J. Marketing for therapists. Tiburon (CA): Jossey-Bass; 1996.
3. The psychiatrist's guide to practice management. Washington, DC: American Psychiatric Association; 1997.
4. US Department of Justice and the Federal Trade Commission. Statements of antitrust policy enforcement in healthcare. 1996. Available at: http://www.usdoj.gov/atr/public/guidelines/1791.htm#CONTNUM_49. Accessed August 30, 2009.
5. The Psychiatrist's managed care primer. Washington, DC: American Psychiatric Association; 1997.
6. Schreter RK. Reorganizing departments of psychiatry, hospitals and medical centers for the 21st century. Psychiatr Serv 1998;49:1429–33.
7. Schreter RK. Earning a living: a blueprint for psychiatrists. Psychiatr Serv 1995; 46:1233–5.
8. Schreter RK. Alternative treatment programs: the psychiatric continuum of care. Psychiatr Clin North Am 2000;23:335–45.
9. Kohen LT, Corrigan JM, Donaldson MS. Institute of Medicine Committee on Quality Health Care in America: to err is human: building a safer health system. Washington, DC: National Academic Press; 2000.
10. Hurd MJ. Productivity and scheduling in a private practice setting. The Behavioral Health Practice Advisor 1996;2:1–4.
11. Ransohoff J. Probing the "mystery" of behavioral case management. Behavioral Health Management 1994;14:29–30.
12. Quality first: better health care for all Americans. Washington, DC: President's Advisory Commission on Consumer Protection and Quality in Health Care Industry; 1998.
13. Epstein AM. The outcomes movement: will it get us where we want to go? N Engl J Med 1990;323:266–9.
14. Lyons J, Howard K, O'Mahoney, et al. The measurement and management of clinical outcomes in mental health. New York: Wiley;1997.
15. American College of Medical Practice Executives: Medical practice management, 2nd edition. Englewood (CO): Medical Group Management Association (MGMA).
16. Kongstevedt PR. Use of data and reports. In: Managed health care handbook. 2nd edition. Gaithersburg (MD): Aspen; 1993.
17. Drucker P. Management tasks, responsibilities, practices. New York: Harper & Row; 1974.
18. Financial Management for Medical Groups. A resource for new and experienced managers. 2nd edition. Englewood (CO): Medical Group Management Association; 2000.

19. Available at: http://en.wikipedia.org/wiki/Medical_malpractice; 2009. Accessed April 15, 2009.
20. Available at: http://en.wikipedia.org/wiki/Errors_and_omissions_insurance; 2009. Accessed April 15, 2009.
21. Available at: http://www.greatamericaninsurance.com/insuranceGlossary.html; 2009. Accessed April 15, 2009.
22. Relman AS. Assessment and accountability: the third revolution in medical care. N Engl J Med 1998;319:1220–2.
23. Schreter RK. Trends in managed care. 2000 edition. Psychiatr Serv 2000:(51);1493–5
24. Schreter RK. Physician service networks and the future for psychiatrists. Psychiatr Serv 1999;50:415–6.
25. Schreter RK. Making due with less: the latest challenge for psychiatry. Psychiatr Serv 2004;55:761–3.
26. Herzlinger R. Market-driven health care: who wins, who loses in the transformation of America's largest service industry. Reading (MA): Addison-Wesley; 1997.

Revenue: Understanding Insurance Reimbursement and CPT Coding in Child and Adolescent Psychiatry

David Berland, MD[a],*, Benjamin Shain, MD, PhD[b,e],
Sherry Barron-Seabrook, MD[c,d]

KEYWORDS

• CPT codes • Fraud • Billing • Reimbursement

Generating revenue from clinical services is essential for practicing child and adolescent psychiatrists. In Part I of this chapter, the authors present a developmental overview of CPT coding, including history, principles, correct coding, and fraud. Part II describes the specialty CPT codes, both psychiatric and other specialties that may be useful to the child and adolescent psychiatrist. Medicare rules allow any physician to use the Evaluation and Management (E/M) Codes. In Part III, the authors discuss them and the complexity of determining the appropriate level of E/M service. Part IV presents examples of different coding approaches for specific services.

PART I: OVERVIEW OF REIMBURSEMENT AND CODING

Revenue is the collected payment for services. Child and adolescent psychiatrists can perform three activities that have revenue potential: research, both basic (grant

[a] Department of Psychiatry, St Louis University School of Medicine, 700 Clayton Road, Suite 103, St Louis, MO 63117, USA
[b] Division of Child and Adolescent Psychiatry, NorthShore University HealthSystem, 777 Park Avenue West, Highland Park, IL 60035, USA
[c] 315 E Northfield Road, Livingston, NJ 07039, USA
[d] Columbia University, College of Physicians and Surgeons, New York, NY, USA
[e] University of Chicago, Chicago, IL, USA
* Corresponding author.
E-mail address: diberland@gmail.com (D. Berland).

Child Adolesc Psychiatric Clin N Am 19 (2010) 89–105
doi:10.1016/j.chc.2009.08.012
1056-4993/09/$ – see front matter © 2010 Elsevier Inc. All rights reserved.

funded) and applied (frequently industry funded); speaking, including teaching; and providing clinical service. This article addresses the process of generating revenue from clinical service. Fee-for-service billing is currently the predominant methodology for generation of the revenue that is needed to pay clinical and support staff as well as practice expenses such as rent, utilities, and other overhead needed to provide care for children, adolescents, and their families coping with mental illness.

The American Medical Association's Current Procedure Terminology—4 (CPT) is the most accepted system used to bill for services. CPT is a list of all health care procedures. Originally designed for Medicare, CPT is now used by private insurance carriers for all age groups. There are thousands of CPT codes—a description of the encounter between patient and provider. The codes are linked to standardized units of work called "Relative Value Units" (RVUs) and standardized units of administrative costs called "Practice Expense."

Of note are legal consequences for misuse of CPT. Specifically, a pattern of erroneous coding may lead to criminal charges of fraud. Conviction carries costly penalties.

Historical Context

Adding private health insurance to benefit packages, employers hoped to recruit and retain workers during World War II. Health care expenses became a significant part of labor negotiations.[1] During World War II, the army surgeon general appointed William Menninger chief psychiatrist to help address the problems of "shell shock" among the military. Dr Menninger increased the number of psychiatrists and psychiatric services. Congress passed the National Mental Health Act of 1946 to fund research and training.

Employer-sponsored health insurance programs funded third-party (private insurance) reimbursement. The combination of the private funding and the federal policy to prioritize mental health treatment stimulated the rapid growth and development of the field of professional mental health services within the health care system.

The enactment of Medicare in the mid 1960s followed by growth in employer-sponsored health coverage in the 1970s (Employee Retirement Income Security Act or ERISA) marked the beginning of the explosion in overall costs of health care. By the mid-1980s, the Health Care Financing Administration (HCFA), the federal agency overseeing Medicare (later renamed Centers for Medicare and Medicaid Services or CMS) adopted the Resource-Based Relative Value Scale (RBRVS).[2] This scale ranked all procedures and professional services in standardized units (RVUs), as a basis for calculating physician payments. In the early 1990s, most private commercial insurance companies adopted parts of this system to standardize physician reimbursement in their networks. CPT-4 provides standardized definitions and numeric codes for all professional services and procedures that physicians perform.

From CPT Codes to Revenue

After the CPT editorial board approves any new procedure, the requesting medical specialty society presents it to the American Medical Association's Relative-value Up-date Committee (RUC).[3] The RUC then recommends a specific place on the RBRVS to CMS. Every year, CMS considers the RUC recommendations and assigns a ranking to the new procedure. (See http://www.cms.hhs.gov/PhysicianFeeSched/ for current ranking of all medical procedures.) Congress sets a number that converts the ranking into dollars. This conversion factor is multiplied by the ranking (expressed in RVUs) to determine actual Medicare payment.

For example, 45 to 50 minutes of interactive psychotherapy in office has a relative value of 3.00. The 2009 conversion factor is about 36. Hence, the Medicare payment is $3.00 \times 36 = \$108.00$.

With this system, Congress can adjust the conversion factor thereby controlling Medicare Part B (physician payments). If tax revenues fall short, Congress can lower the conversion factor and payments to all physicians will be reduced, while preserving the overall RBRVS.

Specialty and Evaluation/Management CPT Codes

The editorial board of CPT assigns a 5-digit CPT code to every medical procedure. There are 2 kinds of CPT procedure codes: specialty and evaluation/management. Child and adolescent psychiatric codes are specialty codes and listed in the Medicine section of CPT, 90800 series. Other specialty codes are located elsewhere in the book; for example, surgical/musculoskeletal (orthopedic surgery) codes are the 20000 series, the surgical/cardiovascular codes are the 33000 series.[4] Organizations may credential certain providers to deliver certain codes (see the section, Private Insurance). For example, a managed behavioral health organization may require its network providers to be psychiatrists, child and adolescent psychiatrists, psychologists, social workers, nurses, or counselors. They credential these providers to use the 90800 codes. Hence, they would not reimburse a pediatrician or family practitioner for these codes.

The second CPT code type is the evaluation and management (E/M) code, 99000 series. These are used for general office visits, emergency room visits, critical care services, home visits, team conferences, and other general medical services that any physician may provide.[4] Many mental health carve-outs do not credential providers to use these codes for outpatients. Hence, they will not pay for them. On the other hand, general medical plans do credential all other physicians to provide these general office visit codes. However, they often do not credential psychiatrists. They "carve-out" that process and contract with mental health organizations to determine which services a provider is qualified to deliver.

Assigning Relative Value Units to CPT Codes

The specialty group that proposes a new code must contact other potentially interested specialty societies to present a relative value for the RUC to recommend to CMS. There are three components to the code's relative value: physician work, practice expense, and professional liability insurance (PLI).

The interested specialty societies survey their members to find out where they think the new code belongs in the RBRVS. The surveys assess the amount of physician work, time, and stress (if the procedure should fail) involved in the service. Respondents rate these factors relative to similar services. For example, 45 to 50 minutes of psychotherapy may be related to an office visit that takes 45 or 50 minutes. If the physician work for that office visit is a 3.0, one would expect the physician work of psychotherapy to be in that neighborhood, say $\pm 15\%$.

Surveys also collect data on the practice expense. Physicians indicate the costs of rent, utilities, equipment, personnel, and so forth used to provide the service. A formula determines the PLI.

These three numbers (Physician work, Practice expense, and PLI) are added together to yield the Relative Value Unit (RVU) that then places the code in an exact location on the RBRVS. As noted previously, the RVU is then multiplied by the conversion factor for payment.

For example, the physician work value for 90811 (interactive psychotherapy, office, 20–30 minutes, with E/M) is 1.48. The practice expense relative value is 0.70. The PLI is 0.04. The sum 2.22 is multiplied by the conversion factor (36) yielding the Medicare payment ($79.92).

Private Insurance

Although the American Medical Association (AMA) created the CPT coding system for Medicare and Medicaid, since the early 1990s, private insurance companies have adopted it as their coding system for payment. However, they select what codes they will cover. In addition, they do not necessarily use the RBRVS. Ignoring the RBRVS, insurance companies arbitrarily set reimbursement rates.

As noted previously, mental health carve-outs further complicate payment issues for child and adolescent psychiatrists. To be paid, the provider must submit a covered CPT code, usually a 90800 code for outpatient visits. It is imperative that the child and adolescent psychiatrist's office communicate directly with each insurer to verify that a specific procedure code is covered and find out the payment rate. Submitting the correct CPT code for a well-documented service does not guarantee payment from a private insurance carrier.

Correct Use of CPT and Fraud

One uses CPT because it is the most widely accepted coding system for payment. When one uses CPT, one must use it correctly. Miscoding and up-coding are examples of fraud and abuse, punishable by fines, imprisonment, or both.

Miscoding in child and adolescent psychiatry could involve coding for an interactive code when not documenting or using play equipment. Another kind of miscoding involves separate billing for services included ("bundled") in one code. For example, billing a 90804 and 90862 is incorrect (fraudulent); the correct code is 90805. In fact, CMS is working to develop software that would detect codes that should never be billed together like 90804 with 90862 or 90806 with 90862, and so forth. This project is called the "National Correct Coding Initiative" (NCCI) and has found more than 500,000 code edits. This problem has much greater potential in other medical specialties. A newer initiative, "Medically Unlikely Edits" (MUE) wants to capture codes that should not be billed on the same day. For example, only one psychotherapy code per patient per day can be submitted.[5]

Up-coding refers to billing a higher level of service than what was provided and usually applies to the E/M codes. Billing an inpatient follow-up visit as a 99233 while only documenting services for a 99232 would be up-coding. (E/M services are discussed in detail later in this article.) An example of up-coding for the 90800 series codes is providing 35 minutes of psychotherapy with E/M and coding that as 90807.

Penalties for fraud and abuse may require payment of damages up to three times the amount of the claim and mandatory penalties of $5,000 to $10,000 per claim, regardless of the size of the claim.[6]

PART II: THE PSYCHIATRY CODES (90800 SERIES) AND OTHER SPECIALTY CODES
Background

In the early 1990s, all mental health practitioners (psychiatrists, psychologists, and social workers, as well as other master's level therapists and nurse practitioners) used three CPT codes for coding individual psychotherapies: 90842 (75–80 minutes), 90843 (20–30 minutes), and 90844 (45–50 minutes). This common usage led to questions about the difference in the work value of the psychotherapy among the different specialties.

In 1995, believing that the psychiatrist's work was fundamentally different from others, the American Psychiatric Association (APA) challenged the assigned work values of the codes. As a result, at the congressionally mandated 5-year review of the codes, CMS replaced the 3 timed individual psychotherapy codes with 24 new psychotherapy codes, based not only on time, but also on the presence or absence of E/M services and the place where the service was rendered. The APA and American Academy of Child and Adolescent Psychiatry (AACAP), as well as the American Psychological Association, National Association of Social Workers, and American Nurse's Association surveyed these codes. Survey results lacked face validity, so the RUC accepted a mathematical model to generate work values for these codes. CMS adopted them in 1999. Controversy regarding these work values continued and these codes are scheduled to be reviewed again in the 5-year review of 2010.

Psychiatric Diagnostic or Evaluative Interview Procedure Codes

There are two CPT codes—90801 and 90802—that describe psychiatric diagnostic or evaluative interview. The psychiatric diagnostic interview examination (90801) includes the history, a mental status examination and disposition, communication with family members or other sources, and ordering, as well as medical interpretation of laboratory or other medical diagnostic studies. In certain circumstances, other informants may be seen in lieu of the patient. The interactive psychiatric diagnostic interview examination (90802) is typically done with children but may be used for an adult who cannot communicate effectively verbally. The interactive evaluation involves the use of physical aids, such as toys or nonverbal communication devices to achieve therapeutic interaction between a clinician and the patient.[4]

Any medical or nonmedically trained health care provider who performs a psychiatric diagnostic procedure may use these codes. Time is not part of the descriptor, but based on provider surveys from 1995, 90801 usually takes 60 minutes of intraservice time (face-to-face), 10 minutes of preservice time, and 55 minutes of postservice time for a total time of 125 minutes. The interactive diagnostic code, 90802, was not surveyed. An expert panel estimated about 75 minutes of face-to-face time with 15 minute of preservice time and 80 minutes of postservice time for a total time of 170 minutes.

These codes do not place any restrictions on how many times they may be used for an evaluation of a patient; however, third-party carriers frequently allow only a one-time use of the code for an individual evaluation. Whereas a comprehensive evaluation of an adult may be completed within a single interview,[7] a comprehensive evaluation of the child or adolescent requires several sessions to complete.[8]

Other Diagnostic Testing Procedure Codes

There are several other diagnostic testing procedures, mostly done by psychologists, but psychiatrists may also use them. These codes are the psychological testing codes (96101 to 96103), neuropsychological testing codes (96118 to 96120), the neurobehavioral status examination (96116), and the developmental testing codes (96110 to 96111). Situations in which these codes may be used include computerized testing for attention problems, other computerized evaluation and testing, and developmental screening checklists and assessments. Some of these tests require specific qualifications for use; but many, especially the computerized tests, do not.

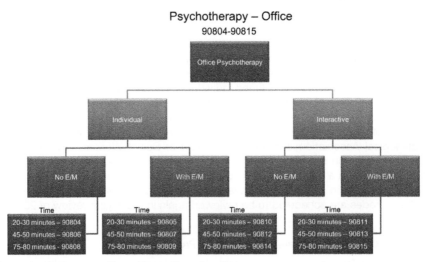

Fig. 1. Psychotherapy office visits coding algorithm.

Not all insurance carriers reimburse for psychological testing. Developmental pediatricians commonly use the developmental testing codes. A physician may bill an E/M code along with the developmental testing codes.

CMS introduced the bundled individual psychotherapy codes in 1996 as G-codes to capture the difference between medical and nonmedical providers.[9] These codes came into effect in 1999 and are based on the following parameters: face-to-face time with the patient (20–30 minutes; 45–50 minutes; 75–80 minutes); site of service (office vs facility, inpatient or residential); presence or absence of E/M services; and type of therapy (verbal insight, supportive, cognitive behavioral vs interactive) (**Figs. 1** and **2**).

Only physicians, nurses, or physician assistants can use E/M codes. The E/M time is *in addition to* the psychotherapy service. The provider must document both the E/M

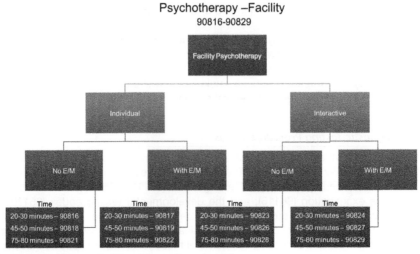

Fig. 2. Psychotherapy facility visits coding algorithm.

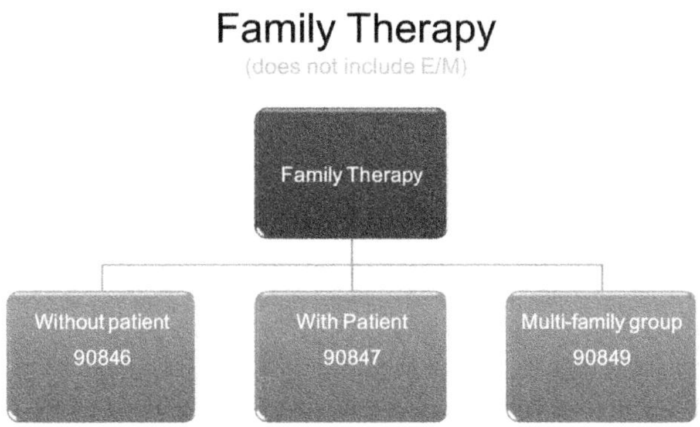

Family Therapy

(does not include E/M)

Family Therapy

| Without patient | With Patient | Multi-family group |
| 90846 | 90847 | 90849 |

Fig. 3. Family therapy visits coding algorithm.

service and the psychotherapy service provided at the visit. E/M services include medical diagnostic evaluation including diagnosis of comorbid medical disorders; medication management; and vital signs such as blood pressure, pulse, height, or weight. To determine the correct code for an individual psychotherapy service, the provider must determine if the procedure is verbal or interactive, does or does not include E/M services, length of time for the service, and where the service was delivered.

Family and Group Therapy Codes

There are specific CPT codes to report family therapy and group therapy. There are 3 family therapy codes: (1) the identified patient is not present (90846), (2) the identified patient is present (90847), and (3) multifamily groups (90849) (**Fig. 3**). The identified patient is billed for the code. E/M services are not included in these codes, but may be bundled in the near future.

There are two group therapy codes: one for standard verbal groups (90853) and another for an interactive, play group, typically done with children (90857). The RVU of the group codes is about one-third of the value for a 45- to 50-minute psychotherapy code without E/M. Again, E/M services are not included in these codes, but that could change. Each participant in the group is billed with the group therapy code and the service must be documented in each participant's medical record (**Fig. 4**).

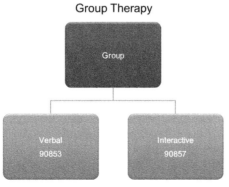

Group Therapy

Group

| Verbal | Interactive |
| 90853 | 90857 |

Fig. 4. Group therapy visits coding algorithm.

Other Psychiatric Services/Procedures Codes

Other useful codes for psychiatrists included pharmacologic management (90862), interpretation to the family (90887), electroconvulsive therapy (90870), review of psychiatric records (90885), and preparation of a report for nonlegal or consultation purposes (90889).

Each insurance carrier has its own rules regarding reimbursement for services provided. An established RVU and acceptance by CMS does NOT guarantee that a third-party payer will cover the service.

Documentation

Documentation requirements for the psychiatric codes have not been specified. At a minimum, the following points are recommended: date and type of service rendered, the person(s) present at the session, mental status of the identified patient, types of interventions used, E/M services provided, diagnosis, and, of utmost importance, a legible medical record.[9]

Miscellaneous Codes

The physician may use any of the codes in the CPT manual as long as the described procedure is performed and documented. However, insurance companies may not reimburse codes unless they have specifically credentialed the physician to perform that service. Examples of miscellaneous codes that may be applicable to psychiatrists include prolonged services (99354 to 99359), care plan oversight (99374 to 99380), medical team conferences (99367), telephone services (99441 to 99443) and polysomnography (95805 to 95811).

PART III: EVALUATION AND MANAGEMENT CODES

E/M codes describe services rendered during a patient visit. These general codes are designed to be used by physicians of all specialties (as well as nurses and physician assistants). The codes should not be confused with psychiatry codes (908xx series), some of which are bundled with evaluation and management as part of the service.

E/M codes are divided into a number of code families depending on the setting and type of service. Examples are office, new patient (99201 to 99205); office, established patient (99211 to 99215); initial hospital or partial hospital (99221 to 99223). Most of the families include either three codes (most inpatient families) or five codes (most outpatient families) codes with the fifth digit determining the level of service.

Determination of Level of Service

The level of service within a code family determines third party payment for that code. However, determination of the fifth digit, as described by the CPT Manual and further explained by CMS, may often be a complex undertaking.

Seven components determine the level of service: history, examination, medical decision making, counseling, coordination of care, nature of presenting problem, and time. Of these, history, examination, and medical decision making are considered to be key components. A notable exception occurs if counseling and coordination of care make up greater than 50% of the face-to-face time (outpatients) or floor time (inpatients) of the visit. Under those circumstances, the clinician may use time to determine the level of service.

As examples, **Tables 1** and **2** list the minimum requirements for the key elements OR time, when appropriate, for the code families 9920x (office visit for new patient) and 9921x (office visit for established patient). For new patients, most of the code

Table 1
Level of coding for office visit, new patient

Code	History	Examination	Medical Decision Making	Time,[a] min
99201	Problem focused	Problem focused	Straightforward	10
99202	Expanded problem focused	Expanded problem focused	Straightforward	20
99203	Detailed	Detailed	Low complexity	30
99204	Comprehensive	Comprehensive	Moderate complexity	45
99205	Comprehensive	Comprehensive	High complexity	60

Select highest code that meets criteria for all three of history, examination, and medical decision making, unless time criteria met (see the section "Counseling and coordination of care").

[a] Time is an alternative criterion for determining level of service when counseling or coordination of care make up greater than 50% of the visit.

families require that all three of the key elements meet the standard for a particular level of service. For established patients, only two of three of the key elements are needed (see the CPT Manual for details for all of the code families).[4]

Requirements for Key Elements

History

History consists of four components: chief complaint (always required); history of present illness; review of systems; and past, family, and social history (PFSH).

History of present illness (HPI) is a description of the development of the patient's present illness from the first sign and/or symptom or from the previous encounter to the present. Elements of HPI may include location, quality, severity, duration, timing, context, modifying factors, and associated signs and symptoms. A *brief* HPI consists of one to three elements of the HPI. An *extended* HPI consists of at least four elements of the HPI or the status of at least three chronic or inactive conditions.

Review of systems (ROS) includes pertinent information from 13 CPT-defined body systems. A *problem pertinent* ROS inquires about the system directly related to the problem(s) identified in the HPI. An *extended* ROS inquires about the system directly related to the problem(s) identified in the HPI plus one to eight additional systems. A

Table 2
Level of coding for office visit, established patient

Code	History	Examination	Medical Decision Making	Time,[a] min
99211			Minimal	5
99212	Problem focused	Problem focused	Straightforward	10
99213	Expanded problem focused	Expanded problem focused	Low complexity	15
99214	Detailed	Detailed	Moderate complexity	25
99215	Comprehensive	Comprehensive	High complexity	40

Select highest code that meets criteria for at least two of three of history, examination, and medical decision making, unless time criteria met.

[a] Time is an alternative criterion for determining level of service when counseling or coordination of care make up greater than 50% of the visit.

Table 3
Type of history

HPI	ROS	PFSH	Type
Brief	N/A	N/A	Problem focused
Brief	Problem pertinent	N/A	Expanded problem focused
Extended	Extended	Pertinent	Detailed
Extended	Complete	Complete	Comprehensive

Abbreviations: HPI, history of present illness; ROS, review of symptoms; N/A, non-applicable; PFSH, past, family, and social history.

complete ROS inquires about the system(s) directly related to the problem(s) identified in the HPI plus at least nine additional body systems. A general statement, such as "compete review of systems is otherwise negative," may be substituted for individual documentation of negative findings for each body system.

Past history includes information about past illness and injury as well as treatment. Family history includes information on medical events and illness in close relatives. Social history includes relevant social factors such as marital status, education, and occupational background. A *pertinent* PFSH is a review of the history area(s) directly related to the problem(s) identified in the HPI (need item from any area). A *complete* PFSH is a review of two (established patient) or all three (new patient) of the PFSH history areas.

Table 3 puts together the results of HPI, ROS, and PFSH to determine the type of history. Chief complaint is not included in the table because it is always required.

Examination

The examination may be a general multisystem examination or 1 of 11 CPT-defined single-system examinations, which includes a psychiatric examination.[10] **Table 4** lists the elements of a single-system psychiatric examination.[11] **Box 1** lists the types of single-system examinations.

Table 4
Psychiatric examination

System/Body Area	Elements of Examination
Constitutional	• At least three vital signs (may be measured and recorded by ancillary staff): • General appearance of patient, eg,
Musculoskeletal	• Assessment of muscle strength and tone (eg, flaccid, cog wheel, spastic) with notation of any atrophy and abnormal movements • Examination of gait and station
Psychiatric	• Speech • Thought process • Associations • Abnormal or psychotic thoughts • Judgment and insight • Orientation • Recent and remote memory • Attention span and concentration • Language • Fund of knowledge • Mood and affect

Box 1	
Types of single-system examinations	
Examination Elements	**Examination Type**
One to five elements identified by a bullet	Problem focused
At least six elements identified by a bullet	Expanded problem focused
At least nine elements identified by a bullet	Detailed
Every element identified by a bullet in each box with a shaded border and at least one element in each box with an unshaded border	Comprehensive

Medical decision making

Medical decision making is divided into three areas: number of diagnoses or manage-ment options; amount or complexity of data reviewed; and risk of complication, morbidity, or mortality.

The number of diagnoses or management options is based on the number or types of problems addressed during the encounter, the complexity of establishing a diag-nosis, and/or the management decisions. Other indicators include that the problem is undiagnosed, the number or types of tests ordered, the need for consultation, and that the problem is worsening.

Amount and/or complexity of data to be reviewed includes factors such as the types of diagnostic tests ordered, review of old medical records (must document the rele-vant findings), history from other sources (must document the relevant findings), and discussion of test results with physician who interpreted the test.

Risk of significant complications, morbidity, and/or mortality is based on risks asso-ciated with the presenting problem, diagnostic procedure, and the possible manage-ment options. The highest level of risk in any one of these categories determines the overall risk. **Table 5** provides examples of risk for various problems, tests, and management options. Note that prescription medication management is at least moderate risk and management of medications requiring intensive monitoring for possible toxicity, such as atypical antipsychotics and antidepressants, is high risk.

Table 6 brings together the three areas to determine the type of medical decision making.

Counseling and coordination of care

The physician may use time as the determining factor of the level of code if the combi-nation of counseling and coordination of care is more than 50% of the time of the encounter. Counseling is not psychotherapy, but rather education regarding illness, tests, and treatment options, including obtaining consent, discussing prognosis, and giving treatment alternatives. Coordination of care includes speaking with team members, outside and past providers, and family members.

The time of the encounter for an outpatient is the amount of time that is spent face-to-face with the patient or a family member. For an inpatient or partial hospital patient, time is the time on the unit doing any activity devoted to the care of the patient in question. CPT chose these parameters because they were considered the most easily and reli-ably measured. Any activity, including counseling or coordination of care, that takes place outside of face-to-face with an outpatient or on the unit (floor time) with an inpa-tient or partial hospital patient is considered to be a pre- or post-time activity. Pre- and post-time activities, such as making phone calls later in the day from the office, are ex-pected aspects of the service for a particular code and have already been factored into

Table 5 Examples of risk			
Presenting Problem(s)	**Diagnostic Procedure(s) Ordered**	**Management Option(s) Selected**	**Level of Risk**
One self-limited or minor problem	Lab testing requiring venipuncture; EKG; urinalysis	Rest; gargles	*Minimal*
Two or more self-limited or minor problems; one stable chronic illness; acute uncomplicated illness	Lab test requiring arterial puncture	OTC drugs; PT; OT	*Low*
One or more chronic illnesses with mild exacerbation, progression, or side effects	Fluid from body cavity	Prescription drug management	*Moderate*
One or more chronic illnesses with severe exacerbation, progression, or side effects	Endoscopy	Drug therapy requiring intensive monitoring for toxicity	*High*

Abbreviations: EKG, electrocardiogram; OT, occupational therapy; OTC, over the counter; PT, physical therapy.

the work value assigned to a code. Time spent doing these activities DOES NOT count toward total encounter time or time spent in counseling or coordination of care.

Documentation for the E/M codes needs to include the length of time of the encounter and the time spent in counseling and coordination of care, as well as a brief description of the counseling and/or coordination of care activities.

Rational Schemes for Determination of Level of Service

As illustrated previously, determination of a single code may require consultation with a vast number of rules and tables. To simplify this task, many physician practices use a small number of codes for the large majority of patient visits. One result is everyone becomes comfortable with those few codes. The temptation, however, is still high to choose codes by guessing based on a several word description on a superbill. Even when guesses are correct, the required elements may not be included in the visit

Table 6 Type of medical decision making			
Number of Diagnoses or Management Options	**Amount or Complexity of Data Reviewed**	**Risk of Complication, Morbidity, or Mortality**	**Type**
Minimal	Minimal or none	Minimal	Straightforward
Limited	Limited	Low	Low complexity
Multiple	Moderate	Moderate	Moderate complexity
Extensive	Extensive	High	High complexity

Select the highest type that includes two of three elements met or exceeded.

documentation. A common practice is to "down code," choosing a lower level of service than what is estimated. This practice does not solve the problem of incomplete documentation and may also result in a significant reduction of revenue compared with using the proper code.

Most visits fit one or more of three patterns, each with its own driving force for coding: problem-oriented, monitoring-oriented, and team-oriented/psychoeducation-oriented. All three of the simplified approaches represent correct coding. Some visits fit more than one pattern. Under those circumstances, the clinician may choose the approach, presumably either the easier one or the one that has greater reimbursement.

Problem-oriented visits

Problem-oriented visits are visits that are required for an acute problem or an acute exacerbation of a chronic problem, such as an emergency outpatient visit or an initial hospital inpatient visit, or are routinely scheduled visits requiring managing an unstable problem as a major part of the work. Medical decision making should be the driving determinant of the level of service for these codes. The level of medical decision making may be quickly inferred by comparing the visit to the child and adolescent psychiatry clinical vignettes at the end of the CPT Manual.[4] These vignettes are highly intuitive, unlike much of the rest of the E/M section. Required elements of history and/or physical examination must still be present but just need to be geared to the level already determined by the medical decision making.

Monitoring-oriented visits

These are scheduled, return visits. The patient may be completely stable, with the visit used for planning and troubleshooting. There may be relatively minor problems that are easily handled. Medical decision making is likely to be at a low level, but codes for these visits generally require only two out of three of history, physical examination, and medical decision making. As a result, the level of the code may be determined by the highest level of history and physical examination needed (and performed/documented) for proper monitoring.

Team-oriented and psychoeducation-oriented visits

These visits occur in team settings, such as inpatient or partial hospital care, in an office setting when most of the visit is spent coordinating care with family members or other professionals, or when most of the visit is spent explaining symptoms, diagnosis, prognosis, testing, or treatment with the patient or family member. What drives the coding of these visits is that counseling and/or coordination of care makes up greater than 50% of the overall time for the visit. Time for an outpatient visits is face-to-face time with a patient or family member and time for a hospital visit is time on the hospital unit devoted to activities in the care of the particular patient. Time determines the level of service and the rules and charts for history, physical examination, and medical decision making are not used.

Coding for Consultation Services

CPT codes for consultations allow physicians to bill for evaluation services requested by a third party. (As this article goes to press, a proposed elimination of the CPT consultation codes is being considered. If this proposal is approved, the clinician should use other E/M codes to report these services.) These codes give psychiatrists the opportunity to bill for the additional work required for a consultation compared with a standard psychiatric evaluation. Since 2006, however, there are fewer types of consultation codes, and requirements for billing a consultation are more stringent.

A consultation is defined as a "type of service provided by a physician whose opinion or advice regarding an evaluation and/or management of a specific problem is requested by another physician or appropriate source" (p.14).[4] The consultant should have more expertise in the specific problem or situation than the requesting provider.

There are now only two types of consultations: outpatient, for service in an office or other ambulatory facility, using codes 99241 to 99245, and inpatient, for service in an inpatient hospital, nursing facility, or partial hospital, using codes 99251 to 99255. Confirmatory consultation codes and follow-up consultation codes have been discontinued. Confirmatory consultations may be reported using a consultation code when the consultation requirements (see the following section) are met. Other confirmatory consultations as well as follow-up visits may be billed with other appropriate nonconsultation E/M codes.[12]

Consultation requirements

Before the consultation, there is a request from a health care professional for the opinion or advice for the evaluation and/or management of specific problem. The request and reason for consultation must be documented in the charts of the requestor and the consultant. After the consultation, the consultant provides the referrer a written report of findings and recommendations.

The intent of the consultation is to obtain an opinion or advice. The person requesting the consultation must also be able to act on the advice. For example, an emergency room physician sending a patient to an outpatient provider or a psychologist requesting a medication evaluation are transfers of care, not consultations, because the requesting providers cannot act on the consultant's recommendations. A consultation may, however, be followed immediately by the consultant assuming care of the patient for a specific problem.

Example situations

Situation 1: The originating physician is unsure of how to treat and requests someone with expertise (the performing physician) for advice. The patient returns to the originating physician and the performing physician may bill a consultation.

Situation 2: The originating physician knows the patient has a problem and that she or he is not the best person to treat the problem. The originating physician asks an expert to treat the patient for the particular problem. This is a transfer of care and may not be billed as a consultation

Situation 3: The originating physician asks the expert for advice. The expert evaluates the patient and then assumes care for the problem in question. This is a consultation followed by treatment.

Special situations

Second opinions initiated by a health care provider may be billed as consultation. Second opinions initiated by the patient or a family member are not consultations, but may be billed with a different evaluation and management ("99xxx") or psychiatric ("908xx") code. Second opinions that are mandated (eg, by third-party payer or hospital) are not covered by Medicare, but may possibly be billed to the mandating entity.

Consults requested by a professional in the same group and the same specialty must include documentation that the consulting professional has expertise in a specific medical area beyond the requesting professional's knowledge. A supervisor may not be asked for consultation.

For inpatient hospital, nursing facility, and partial hospital, each physician may only report a consult code once per stay, even if a new problem develops. For this purpose, physicians of the same specialty AND group are considered the same physician. For outpatients, a consult code may be billed each time a new consultation is requested for the same or different problem even by the same requestor.

PART IV: CODING OPTIONS

Child and adolescent psychiatrists may use either the E/M codes or the psychiatric specialty codes when coding for patient encounters. (Consideration of which categories of code insurance companies cover is often the decisive factor.) For initial evaluations, an initial visit code for a new patient (99205, outpatient or 99233, inpatient) or 90801 and 90802 may be used.

There are several options for coding office visits for pharmacologic management. The most frequently used code is 90862, but the E/M codes may be used as an alternative. Choosing the correct E/M codes is based on the complexity of the situation (as described previously). The 90862 has a relative value between 99212 and 99213, which are low complexity codes. Many child and adolescent psychiatric patients are moderately to highly complex, requiring more than two medications, most of which are not approved for use in children or have Black Box warnings. The higher level E/M codes, 99214 or 99215 provide better options for coding these visits and may be reimbursed at higher rates. Appropriate documentation of services is required when these codes are used. (As noted earlier, as this article goes to press, a proposed elimination of the CPT consultation codes is being considered. If this proposal is approved, the clinician should use other E/M codes to report these services.) The payment caveat bears repeating: insurance companies may not reimburse at all for codes unless they specifically credential the physician to perform that service (**Fig. 5**).

Coding for psychotherapy visits is straightforward (see **Figs. 1** and **2**). The E/M component is very minimal in these visits and is added on to the therapy time requirement. Using modifiers may be helpful. For example, if a patient is seen for psychotherapy for 32 minutes, but then requires a few more minutes for an E/M service,

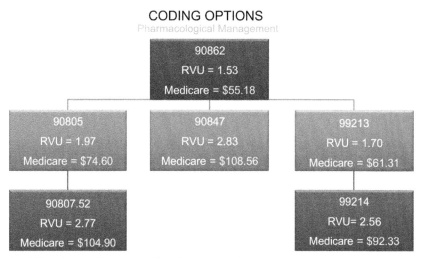

CODING OPTIONS
Pharmacological Management

90862
RVU = 1.53
Medicare = $55.18

90805
RVU = 1.97
Medicare = $74.60

90847
RVU = 2.83
Medicare = $108.56

99213
RVU = 1.70
Medicare = $61.31

90807.52
RVU = 2.77
Medicare = $104.90

99214
RVU= 2.56
Medicare = $92.33

Fig. 5. Office visits coding options for pharmacologic management. Based on 2009 Medicare nonfacility rates.

the code 90807.52 may be used. The .52 modifier means that the procedure was essentially the same as the code descriptor, but was modified slightly. In this instance, the psychotherapy component was shorter than the required 45 to 50 minutes. This modifier can be used with any code.

Coding for prolonged visits may be done by using the prolonged visits codes. For example, if a patient is seen in a crisis situation and the visit takes about 2 hours, then one can use a 90809 (outpatient) or 90822 (inpatient) code and for the additional 40 minutes, use the prolonged services 99354 (outpatient) or 99356 (inpatient) code. The need for the prolonged services must be documented, and third-party payers may require a letter of explanation for the prolonged services.

It is very important to determine the specific procedures third-party carriers will cover. Medicare publishes their payment policies on all the codes for the medical specialties. Insurance carriers vary significantly in their payment policies. Many do not recognize outpatient E/M codes for psychiatric reimbursement, so the psychiatrist is restricted to using the psychiatric procedure codes.

SUMMARY

Correct coding is a necessary skill for all physicians. Psychiatrists must be familiar with both the standard E/M codes that all physicians use to code for office or inpatient visits as well as the psychiatric codes that are specific for psychiatric procedures. Correct coding enables the physician to obtain the best reimbursement for the services rendered. Understanding the coding system and using it appropriately is important to avoid costly medical audits and accusations of fraud and abuse.

As this article goes to press, reimbursement for psychiatric care is rapidly changing. In 2010, mental health parity requires the same limits and benefits (eg, copays, number of visits per calendar year, annual maximum benefit, and so forth) for mental and other medical illnesses. The psychiatric procedure codes are expected to be reviewed by the RUC in the upcoming 5-year review. The current RVUs of the psychiatric procedure codes will be compared with other medical procedure codes. Psychiatric practice has significantly changed since the last 5-year review and the codes are considered to be undervalued. Hopefully this inequality will be rectified. The AACAP and APA are considering a proposal to modify some of the code descriptors. Possibilities exist for developing additional codes that more accurately describe current psychiatric practice. These codes must then be submitted to CPT for approval, surveyed by AACAP and other interested organizations and presented to the RUC for recommendations to CMS, approximately a 2- to 3-year process. These efforts should provide child and adolescent psychiatrists more appropriate coding options for patient care and lead to better reimbursement for the rendered services.

REFERENCES

1. Fein R. Health care reform. Sci Am 1992;46–53.
2. Hsaio WC. The Resource-Based Relative Value Scale: toward the development of an alternative physician payment system. JAMA 1987;258(6):799–802.
3. The American Academy of Pediatrics has produced a survival guide for the CPT-RUC process. Available at: http://www.aap.org/sections/critcare/cptruc processessek.pdf. Accessed June, 2009.
4. Current Procedure Terminology. Professional edition. Chicago: American Medical Association; 2009.
5. Available at: http://www.cms.hhs.gov/MLNProducts/downloads/MCRP_Booklet. pdf. Information about NCCI edits and MUE's. Accessed June, 2009.

6. Baumann L. An introduction to health care fraud and abuse. In: Baumann L, editor. Health care fraud and abuse: practical perspectives. 2nd edition. Arlington (VA): BNA Books; 2007.
7. American Psychiatric Association. Practice guidelines for the psychiatric evaluation of adults, second edition. Am J Psychiatry 2006;163(Suppl 6):3–36.
8. American Academy of Child and Adolescent Psychiatry. Assessment of a child and adolescent. J Am Acad Child Psychiatry 1997;36(Suppl).
9. Schmidt CW, Yowell RK, Jaffe E. The CPT handbook for psychiatrists. 3rd edition. Washington, DC: APA Publishing Press; 2004.
10. Guidelines for documentation of evaluation & management services. Available at: http://www.cms.hhs.gov/MLNProducts/Downloads/1995dg.pdf. 1995. Accessed June, 2009.
11. Guidelines for documentation of evaluation and management services. Available at: http://www.cms.hhs.gov/MLNProducts/Downloads/MASTER1.pdf. 1997. Accessed June, 2009.
12. Federal Register, Part II. Centers for Medicare and Medicaid services, July 13, 2009. p. 33551–4.

The Psychiatric Medical Record, HIPAA, and the Use of Electronic Medical Records

Michael Houston, MD[a,b,*]

KEYWORDS

- Confidentiality • HIPAA • Electronic medical records
- Children • Psychiatry

Whatever, in connection with my professional practice or not, in connection with it, I see or hear, in the life of men, which ought not to be spoken of abroad, I will not divulge, as reckoning that all such should be kept secret.

The Hippocratic Oath

The medical record serves first and foremost as a tool for physicians and other health care providers to document and track their observations, interactions, interventions, and the progress of the patient's disease and treatment. As with other areas of medicine, the purpose and use of the medical record has grown increasingly complex. A patient's record is now used to ensure continuity of care within a multiphysician group or clinic and within large health care systems, such as the Veterans Administration.[1] The record is used to determine and justify diagnoses, billing, and reimbursement. In matters of litigation, it is a legal document serving to determine whether an individual received proper care. Although medical records have long been the source of retrospective research data, as we move into an era of electronic records, the data within each individual's medical record potentially will become part of national system of data exchange allowing real-time analysis of disease trends, treatment use and effectiveness, and drug safety monitoring.

---

[a] Department of Psychiatry and Behavioral Sciences, George Washington University Medical School, Washington, DC, USA
[b] Department of Pediatrics, George Washington University Medical School, Washington, DC, USA
* 4812 Falstone Avenue, Chevy Chase, MD 20815.
E-mail address: mhoustonmd@gmail.com

Child Adolesc Psychiatric Clin N Am 19 (2010) 107–114
doi:10.1016/j.chc.2009.08.011   childpsych.theclinics.com
1056-4993/09/$ – see front matter © 2010 Published by Elsevier Inc.

The psychiatrist and mental health care provider face significant responsibilities when it comes to protecting the confidentiality of their patient's medical information that are mandated by one's professional ethics in addition to state and federal law.[2] In the case of child and adolescent mental health records, there are added concerns regarding confidentiality when one considers the inclusion of family mental health histories and the child or adolescent's particular right to confidentiality that exists above and beyond parental rights.[3]

This article briefly reviews the necessary components of the psychiatric record and issues regarding the confidentiality of mental health records. It also addresses the basic requirements mandated by the Health Insurance Portability and Accountability Act of 1996 (HIPAA). The emerging use of electronic medical records (EMR) is also discussed, with focus primarily on their application within the outpatient practice of child and adolescent psychiatry.

THE PSYCHIATRIC MEDICAL RECORD

The content and purpose of the medical record has and will continue to evolve over time. Within a solo outpatient practice, the medical record has always provided a record of the clinician's observations, interactions, and interventions with an individual patient. Within institutions such as clinics and hospitals, it has served the same purpose while also providing a means of communicating such information among all those involved in an individual's care. Although these remain the primary purposes of the medical record, the record has evolved over time into a legal document that needs to justify that adequate care and information was provided to a patient.[4] The medical record also serves as a resource for quality improvement and for billing and reimbursement issues related to insurers and third party payers, such as Medicaid and Medicare. With the increasing use of EMRs and their potential to incorporate treatment guidelines and access to large databases containing information on treatment outcomes and pharmacologic interactions, the medical record has already started to evolve into a clinical resource of its own that has the potential to vastly improve the quality and efficiency of the care being provided.

Contents of the Psychiatric Medical Record

Within the outpatient practice of child and adolescent psychiatry, there are few, if any, rules that mandate what the individual clinician's records must include or how they should be organized. General guidelines would call for making the record as complete as possible so that it adequately records the work that was done in evaluating, diagnosing, and treating an individual patient. The record should include sections for the patient's personal and financial information. The psychiatric record also includes pertinent personal and administrative information, such as names of parents or guardians, addresses, phone numbers, employer and insurance information, treatment authorizations, consent to treat forms, notification of release of information policies, and record of the actual release of information whether to the patient, consulting clinicians, or to third party payers.

Pertinent clinical information includes the appropriate medical and psychiatric history; initial assessment and diagnostic impressions; an initial treatment plan; and a record of all subsequent visits detailing dates and length of sessions, notable changes in clinical presentation and adjustments to or continuation of the treatment plan, such as refills or new prescriptions, consultations, and other interventions. Clear and adequate documentation that patients and/or their guardians have been informed of the benefits, risks, and potential complications of medications and other therapeutic interventions is important. The medical record should also document the physician's thinking and the actions that she or he decided to take or not to take with regard to suicidal or homicidal thinking and behavior and other high-risk situations.[4]

The level of detail recorded in the psychiatric record is especially pertinent to the child and adolescent psychiatrist, with whom information regarding the patient, their parents and guardians, and other family members is routinely discussed. The guideline here should be one of adequately recording clinically relevant information without jeopardizing the privacy and intimate details of all matters that come to the attention of the physician. As an example, consider the case of a child patient treated in the context of a contentious parental divorce. Although certainly it would make sense to document aspects of the divorce and the parental discord that directly affect the child and your treatment, clinical judgment needs to be used in determining how much of the details of the discord need to be recorded, especially in light of the real possibility of a parent later requesting the clinical record as part of a divorce proceeding. A different level of recording would be indicated when reviewing matters related to suspected physical or sexual abuse.[3]

Detailed process notes, although helpful to a clinician in understanding and tracking the course of therapeutic process, should probably not be kept as part of the patient's standard medical record. Courts and regulatory agencies have indicated that if such records are kept separate and distinct from the medical record, they need not be released under most subpoenas or request for records release and instead are considered the private notes of the clinician. The key factor here is that such notes are kept physically separate from the medical record.[5,6]

With regard to child and adolescent psychiatrists working within hospitals or other institutions, the requirements for what is included in the medical record is generally mandated by the institution, based on requirements of outside accreditation bodies such as the Joint Commission on Accreditation of Healthcare Organizations.[7] According to the type of institution within which a clinician works, the requirements for what is included in the medical record can be quite different and sometimes problematic. For example, a children's medical hospital with both inpatient and outpatient child and adolescent psychiatric services usually have centralized medical record departments that mandate the use of specific forms for reporting outpatient visits and many additional requirements for the documentation of inpatient treatment. This information often becomes part of the child or adolescent's general medical record and could be provided any time his or her medical record is released. In these situations, a clinician must use discretion regarding what information is included in the patient's psychiatric record, so as not to compromise the confidential nature of the relationship between the psychiatrist and patient. Ideally in such institutions, records of mental health treatment encounters, outpatient or inpatient, are kept physically separate from general medical records. The situation is usually different in a freestanding psychiatric facility or residential treatment center where generally extremely detailed record keeping is the norm and adequate safeguards are in place to ensure that inappropriate nondisclosure will not occur.

Legal Issues Related to Psychiatric Medical Records

Despite the passage of the HIPAA of 1996, federal legislation that aimed at ensuring the privacy of protected health care information, most of the legal issues pertaining to psychiatric medical records of children and adolescents are based on state law and hence vary widely. A commonly encountered question is who (child, adolescent, parent, guardian) has access to the record. Here it is not feasible to talk about what most states mandate. One needs to know the state laws and regulations relevant to one's practice, and even then the issues may not be entirely clear. Generally, a custodial parent is permitted access to the psychiatric record of their minor child. In some states, a noncustodial parent may also have rights to review treatment records. Even more complicated is the question of what access a parent may have to treatment records for an adolescent who independently seeks mental health treatment. More complicated still is whether a parent has access to such records when the adolescent independently seeks treatment but a parent is providing reimbursement for the treatment.[8] In such matters it is important to know your individual state's regulations and to use your best clinical judgment, supplemented when necessary by legal consultation.

Technically, medical records, including mental health records, belong to the physician. If employed by an institution, such as a hospital or clinic, the institution owns the record. Patients or their guardians have a right to access the information within those records, and most jurisdictions have statutes that require a physician to provide copies of a patient's medical record within a reasonable period of time and at a reasonable cost covering the materials and time involved in creating a copy.[8]

State laws vary as to how long one must retain a medical or psychiatric record and, at times, the manner in which it should be destroyed. For example, in the state of Maryland, where the author practices, medical records need to be retained for 5 years. In the case of minors, the records need to be retained for 5 years or for 3 years after the patient turns 18 years old, depending on which is longer.[9] In some states, records are required to be kept for as long as 10 years.

Common sense would tell us that records should be legible and that once placed in a chart they should not be altered. If corrections need to be made, it is best to do so by crossing out incorrect material with a single line that does not obscure what was originally written and/or make such corrections with an addendum to a note.

CONFIDENTIALITY UNDER HIPAA

Given the complexity and broad scope of HIPAA, it is easy to forget that the primary purpose of the legislation was to ensure that individuals with preexisting conditions would not be denied health insurance coverage if they changed jobs or if their employers changed insurance. Although this is still an integral part of the legislation, the mental health clinician is more likely to be faced with deciphering the aspect of the regulations that deal with patient privacy and confidentiality. As part of the scope of HIPAA, regulations were enacted after its passage in 1996 to provide protection to an individual's health care information, specifically the electronic exchange of such information, which occurs with electronic claims submission, electronic prescribing, and/or the transfer of patient records by any electronic means, including facsimile and email.

The privacy provisions and regulations set forth under HIPAA apply only to those health care providers and institutions that are considered "covered entities." As a mental health clinician, a simple rule for determining whether you are a covered entity is to review whether in your practice any information regarding patient care, that is, billing, prescriptions, prescriptions preauthorizations, treatment authorizations, and/or patient records, are submitted or transferred by electronic means, such as direct electronic claims submission, facsimile, or email. Although it might be possible for a clinician in solo private practice to avoid any of these activities, it is becoming increasing unlikely as we all become more dependent on these various technologies for the fast and efficient exchange of information.[10,11]

For the small solo or group practice, the administrative regulations that fall under HIPAA do not need to be burdensome. First and foremost is the need to inform patients of what your practice's disclosure policies are; this is usually done by means of a 1- or 2-page document that a patient can review and sign at their first visit. This document should outline the policies regarding the privacy of their health care information. For example, it might spell out that information will not be released without a signed disclosure, except for information required to submit claims and/or other insurance information. The second aspect is to have in place written practice policies regarding individual health care records, such as where the records are stored, who has access to them, and how it is ensured that disclosures are only made appropriately. This is relatively easy to accomplish within a solo practice, but one must be mindful about keeping personal health care information separate from billing and administrative information if one uses employed or contracted individuals for those roles. Within a group practice, or even a large solo practice with several ancillary staff, the physician must also be able to document that the staff has been trained and that adequate and appropriate privacy policies are in place.

One aspect of HIPAA should be kept in mind, especially as it applies to mental health information.[12] HIPAA sets a basic level of regulation regarding the privacy of health information. Included in the legislation is the understanding that information needs to be exchanged regularly between health care professionals involved in an individual patient's treatment. In these situations, a specific signed release of information is not necessary, as the legislation allows for the exchange of clinical information between 2 or more consulting and collaborating health care providers. This is important when one considers the necessity and utility of regularly exchanging information between the child and adolescent psychiatrist and the patient's pediatrician or the exchange of information that would be needed when a patient is hospitalized or needs emergency care. It is important to remember, however, that these guidelines for exchange of information may be preempted by more stringent state laws regarding the release of mental health information.

ELECTRONIC MEDICAL RECORDS

The implementation and use of EMRs has already begun to transform the manner in which health care information is collected, shared, and used. The judicious use and the standardization of EMRs have the potential to greatly increase the efficiency of the delivery of health care services by reducing costs, primarily through elimination of redundancy, and implementing cost-effective evidenced-based treatments.[13,14] If one considers the use of large-scale databases to monitor medication and treatment side effects and safety, EMRs also have the potential to greatly improve the quality and safety of the care. The question remains as to how the widespread implementation of EMRs might affect the provision of mental health care, especially given the customary expectation of a higher level of confidentiality associated with mental health treatment. A challenge for all system-based EMRs is how to insure patient privacy while allowing appropriate accessibility.[15]

Other advantages of using EMRs include streamlining the collection of data through the use of computer-based forms. This might include the use of standardized and validated symptom checklists and the use of short template progress notes. Many systems provide the capacity to efficiently export data to create treatment summaries. If working within a group practice or if employing administrative staff, the ability to assign levels of access to patient information based upon an employee's need to know is an important feature that limits the inappropriate disclosure of information. The integration of electronic prescribing capabilities, in which prescriptions are either faxed or transmitted electronically to the patient's pharmacy, is another clear advantage. The latter generally includes automatic access to databases that can check formulary limitations based on insurer, dosage guidelines, and drug interactions, adding to their capacity to increase efficiency and improve safety.

For the purpose of discussion, it is important to differentiate between EMRs that stand in place of the paper medical record and practice management systems (PMS) that are used to automate patient scheduling and billing. Systems that provide both of these functions within a single program (or those which have an effective electronic interface between the 2 systems) can be quite advantageous by eliminating the need for redundant data entry.

Whether setting up an office as a solo practitioner or within a group practice, adequate time and research needs to be given to selecting the appropriate software and system. As a child and adolescent psychiatrist, the purchase of a fully functional EMR will likely be the largest practice expense exceeding or equaling the cost of the lease of the office. A good, well-functioning system will save time and money, whereas the wrong choice will cost the same in addition to the frustration that will be caused. Before beginning the research, a checklist of the attributes that are necessary and desirable should be created. Many companies offer online demo versions of their software or provide demonstration in the exhibition areas at professional conferences. Even with the best systems, technical support is almost always necessary; therefore it would be wise to consider the availability and cost of such support.

Even at this early stage of evolution, there are numerous software vendors offering EMRs suitable for child and adolescent psychiatrists in small group or solo practice settings. Given the ways in which HIPAA legislation has set standards for encryption of health care information, systems currently marketed generally include the mandated encryptions standards. The format of the EMRs fall into either of 2 models: (1) locally based systems where the software and records are run and stored on computers within the clinician's office and (2) Web-based systems where software and records are stored on a centralized computer server owned by the vendor and accessed via an Internet browser. Either type may offer similar features, such as the ability to customize forms, interaction with dictation systems, and interoperability with the office's PMS. Although local-based systems often have higher startup costs ($2000–$20,000), with adequate technical support they can be highly customizable and have the clear advantage that data (the patient's record) remain in the clinician's office and are theoretically more secure.[16] Disadvantages of the local system include that without adequate backup, data can be lost or become unavailable for some period of time as a result of local computer malfunction or other catastrophes. Web-based EMRs have lower startup costs, as the physician user or clinic pays monthly for access and use of the Web-based software. They also have the advantage, should it be needed, that patient records are accessible from any computer connected to the Internet. Although data are stored in secure servers and are routinely backed up, the involvement of a third party (ie, the information technology vendor) in the management of the data creates a potential for breaches in security and the potential loss of confidentiality. One could argue that these same threats exist in some way for local computer systems and for that matter for paper records also. Another issue to be considered and negotiated with the Web-based system is what happens to the data and the records when the clinician terminates the contract or switches to another vendor. Most companies with allow the export of data either in the form of printed records or through a commonly used database, such as Microsoft Excel, before destroying the records that have been created.

FINAL CONSIDERATIONS

Given that confidentiality is paramount to the psychiatric medical record, finding a means to safeguard the information in the office's records needs to be an ongoing concern. In an office with paper records, the issues become the locks on the office door and the security of the filing cabinet. With EMRs, the issues are even more significant when one considers that records of your patients could be compromised with indiscriminate use of a computer password or the theft of a laptop or backup computer drive. Computer systems need to be secured by the use of locked physical access, adequate encryption, and suitably complex and indecipherable passwords. Within the physician's office and administrative areas, the use of privacy screens on computer monitors that might be within sight of patients reduce the possibility of inadvertent disclosures much in the way that one would safeguard a paper appointment calendar.

The increased use of EMRs is being emphasized as an important aspect of health care reform. The wide-scale adoption of EMRs indeed promises to increase the ease with which information can be shared among providers, thereby improving the efficiency of health care delivery by reducing redundancy, simplifying billing, and improving quality and safety. On the other hand, concerns regarding potential threats to the security and privacy of patients' mental health information within large databases designed for the ready exchange of information have been appropriately raised by mental health providers[15] and represent significant implementation challenges as child and adolescent psychiatry moves further into the digital era.

REFERENCES

1. Luo J. Electronic medical records. Prim psychiatry 2006;13(2):20–3.
2. Petrila J. Medical records confidentiality: issues affecting mental health and substance abuse systems. Drug Benefit Trends 1999;11(3):6–10.
3. Faille L, Clair M, Penn J. Special risk management issues in child and adolescent psychiatry. Psychiatr Times 2007;24(8).
4. Practice management for early career psychiatrists. chapter 24, medical records American Psychaitric Association. 2006. Available at: http://www.psych.org/Main Menu/PsychiatricPractice/ManagingYourPractice/PracticeManagementHandbookfor ECPs.aspx. Accessed October 19, 2009.
5. Vanderpool D. Do patients have access to therapy or personal notes. (American Psychiatric Association). Psychiatr News 2008;43(8):24.
6. Psychotherapy notes provision of the Health Insurance Portability and Accountability Act (HIPAA) privacy rule, 2002. Policy statement of the American Psychiatric Association Resource Document, APA Doc Ref No. 200201.
7. 1999 Comprehensive Accreditation Manual for Hospitals. Joint Commission of Accreditation of Healthcare Organizations. p. IM 7.1–7.8
8. Miller R, Hutton R. Healthcare information. In: Miller R, editor. Problems in healthcare law. 8th edition. Gaithersburg (MD): Aspen Publishers; 2000. p. 532–79.
9. Moffet B. Document retention policies, Mid-Atlantic health law topics. Topics 2005. Available at: http://www.gfrlaw.com/pubs/GordonPubDetail.aspx?xpST= PubDetail&pub=313. Accessed October 19, 2009.
10. Malek L, Krex B. HIPAA and mental health information: know the law. In Confidence 2002;10(11):1–2.
11. HIPAA compliance: introduction for AACAP Members, The American Academy of Child & Adolescent Psychiatry. Available at: http://www.aacap.org/cs/root/

legislative_action/hipaa_compliance_introduction_to_aacap_members. Accessed October 19, 2009.
12. Appelbaum P. Privacy in psychiatric treatment: threats and responses. Am J Pschiatry 2002;159(11):1809–18.
13. Institute of Medicine. Crossing the quality chasm: a new health system for the 21st century. Washington, DC: National Academy of Sciences; 2003.
14. Lawlor T, Barrows E. Behavioral health electronic medical record. Psychiatr Clin North Am 2008;31:95–103.
15. Mandl D, Szolovits P, Kohane I. Public standards and patients' control: how to keep electronic medical records accessible but private. BMJ 2001;322:283–7.
16. Bergeron B. Small practice EMR's. MedGenMed 2004;6(1):e17.

Ethics and Risk Management in Administrative Child and Adolescent Psychiatry

Adrian Sondheimer, MD[a,b],*

KEYWORDS

- Ethics • Risk management • Children
- Adolescents • Psychiatry • Administration

It is appropriate that the recent edition of one of the most esteemed child and adolescent psychiatry (CAP) texts places its content between an introductory article on ethics and a closing forensic subsection devoted to risk management.[1] This sequence suggests that the editors understand that ethical considerations underlie all medical and psychiatric practice, and that risk management (RM) anticipates the pitfalls of not taking these ethical standards, considerations, and guidelines sufficiently seriously. Notwithstanding the close relationship between the two, however, ethics and RM are two distinct areas that warrant separate scrutiny, although their relationship also merits investigation.

Ethics is a system of inquiry that focuses on distinguishing rightful from wrongful behaviors and encourages most helpful or least harmful comportment among individuals and groups.[2,3] RM also encourages good or best behaviors toward individuals and groups, by attempting to reduce risks to levels acceptable to society. In contrast to ethics, however, RM explicitly encourages such behaviors to spare individuals and groups from excessive expenditures and future grief in the legal arena.[4]

In the medical context, considerations of ethics and RM practices aim to result in at least adequate patient care.[5] Thus the 2 topics are commonly conflated. Also, clinical decision-making, RM decisions should be based, at least in part, on an ethical reasoning process. In this article, each subject is approached initially as a separate entity. Subsequently, the manner in which ethical thinking informs RM practices is reviewed.

---

[a] 451 West End Avenue, Suite 2H, New York, NY 10024, USA
[b] Division of Child and Adolescent Psychiatry, UMDNJ-New Jersey Medical School, Newark, NJ, USA
* 451 West End Avenue, Suite 2H, New York, NY 10024.
E-mail address: adriansondheimer@aol.com

Child Adolesc Psychiatric Clin N Am 19 (2010) 115–129
doi:10.1016/j.chc.2009.08.002
1056-4993/09/$ – see front matter © 2010 Elsevier Inc. All rights reserved.

ETHICS

Ethics is a discipline that examines the rightness or wrongness of human behaviors and the moral basis for the distinction. A moral consensus reflects behavioral norms within societies; moral behaviors, in contrast to immoral ones, are actions promoting individuals' and societal welfare. Philosophic ethics rests on theoretic approaches and constructs that include principles, postulated "virtuous" character traits, and theories, such as beneficence, trustworthiness, empathy, (absolutist) deontology, and (relativist) utilitarianism.[6] Applied ethics uses these approaches and incorporates them into reflections devoted to specific disciplines. Thus, ethics applied to the fields of medicine and psychiatry (a medical specialty) yields medical ethics and psychiatric ethics.

Medicine and psychiatry are professions that have evolved. Given advances in mores, knowledge, and technology in both disciplines, ethical quandaries have grown more complex. For example, the last century has witnessed a shift in medicine from paternalism to an emphasis on patient autonomy and informed consent; from reliance on support derived from close physician-patient relationships to dependence on designer pharmaceuticals and technical equipment; and from diagnostic guesswork based on gross signs and symptoms to objective analyses of subcellular and genetic structures. Independent of era, the categories of basic ethical quandaries remain unchanged, for example, confidentiality, autonomy, boundaries, and not doing harm. The contemporary settings in which these concerns confront clinical physicians and physician administrators, however, have become progressively more complicated.

Children and Ethics

The work of child and adolescent psychiatrists commonly centers on young people. Children ordinarily differ from adults in physique, language mastery, range of knowledge, and their ability to maneuver through the world on their own. With time, mastery improves, and professionals who work with children must be aware of continuous maturational and developmental change. Children's developmental immaturities and their consequences are ever present, however, and ethical considerations applied to children therefore involve factors additional to those that apply to adults.[7] Thus, a child's decisions about medical treatments may be compromised by cognitive immaturity, resulting in the physician's acknowledgment that the child's preferences usually require approval or rejection by responsible adult guardians. Adult guardians supply pertinent and necessary information about the child to the physician; in turn, the guardians expect information about diagnosis and treatment from the practitioner. In addition, it is often the guardians' role and responsibility to institute and maintain their children's treatment. Handling concerns surrounding confidentiality and information exchange involves several protagonists in addition to the individual child patient, and may be considerably more complicated than when dealing with competent adults. Along various developmental parameters, 3-year-old children and 17-year-old young people differ enormously from each other, and they both differ from children along the continua of ages dividing them. Consequently, CAP practitioners must be aware of the developmental attainments of each individual child in their care when considering confidentiality and autonomy concerns.

Ethics and Administration

Cardinal principles, often considered foundations for ethical analyses, include beneficence ("doing good"), nonmaleficence ("avoiding harm"), autonomy ("rights of individual"), and justice ("treating all equally").[8] They can be applied to cases involving individuals and large groups. The latter could include unit staffs, hospital personnel, research cohorts, defined demographic populations, behavioral health organizations, and entire countries. CAP administrators have responsibility for the welfare of individual patients directly or indirectly in their care, and are equally responsible for small or large groups of individuals. Thus, for example, shifting personnel from one site to another, limiting availability of medicines in a hospital formulary, enforcing inclusion and exclusion criteria in a treatment research study, and creating a hierarchy of diagnoses deemed worthy or unworthy of insurance coverage, are decisions affecting groups of different sizes. Rigorous ethical reasoning and analysis[9] should underlie the decisions in these scenarios, identical to the manner in which that process is used in cases affecting individual patients.

RM

RM is a structured administrative approach designed to minimize uncertainty and, to the extent possible, avoid litigation.[10] In the medical context, whereas ethics focuses on the promotion of patients' welfare, RM concentrates on sparing individual practitioners, agencies, institutions, and corporations the emotional and financial tribulations attendant to the receiving end of malpractice and liability lawsuits. It is understood that treating patients entails the certainty of professional errors. Depending on the severity of the errors, extent of the injured persons' anger, and degrees of negligence attributed to the agency or practitioner, a small percentage of such errors result in lawsuits.[11] In the United States, patients are enti-tled to seek compensation for injuries caused by errors in medical treatments and procedures. Medical care institutions and practitioners must, in turn, anticipate such occurrences. They reduce their exposure and promote their opportunities for continuing in practice by engaging in activities designed to diminish the occurrence of errors, hence RM.

RM involves a sequence of activities: risk identification and assessment; creation of objectives; development of strategies; and institution of policies and efforts to mitigate identified risks using available resources. Potential strategies could include: elimi-nating risk possibility (eg, a priori not offering a specific service); transferring risk (eg, purchasing insurance; outsourcing procedures); reducing chances of risk (eg, education of staff personnel); and accepting a risk level (eg, provision of average quality of typical mainstream medical care; budgeting for malpractice and liability insurance coverage).[12]

Quality assessment and improvement is a systematic process integral to RM. Ideally, the identification of risks results in improvement of institutional and personal value via policy creation and enactment. These policies should be evidence based, tailored to specific risks, flexibly adaptable, open to new data, and capable of change. Potential pitfalls to guard against in this process include excessive reliance on risk avoidance, thus eliminating an institution's or practitioner's willingness to provide care; potential inflexibility of enacted procedures, thus inhibiting adaptive responses to new challenges; and unwillingness to expend costly resources of time and money on the identification and assessment process. Such short-sighted choices could decrease the viability of the enterprise or practice for the longer term.

RM and Medicine

Given individual variation among human beings, it is expected that provision of medical care is accompanied periodically by outcomes that are poorer than hoped for, innocent mistakes, or frank injuries to patients. These sequelae are expected costs of medical interventions; the goal of RM is to identify those that could be prevented. For example, an adequate staff/patient ratio would likely ensure suitable care for the majority of hospitalized patients; by contrast, an inadequate number of personnel would predictably lead to ignorance of the needs of some patients, resulting in poorer outcomes if not harm. Medical care and treatment lead at times to "complications," which can take different forms. Treatment with medications not infrequently results in patients experiencing disturbing side effects; poor treatment results can be the consequence of well-intentioned and well-provided care (as illustrated by the quip "The operation was a success but the patient died"); and some complications result from institutional, staff, or physician negligence, which reflects failure on the part of those responsible to provide adequate medical care. This last scenario most commonly leads to malpractice litigation, the bane of and impetus for RM.

Malpractice

For a legal finding of medical malpractice to occur, it must be established that: the alleged malfeasor had a duty to care for the patient; the accused was derelict in that duty; the patient consequently experienced harm or injury; and the accused's actions or inactions were the proximate cause (ie, were the direct precipitants of the harm or injury).[13,14] Although some derelictions may seem self-evident, because of legitimate differences in perspective among the protagonists, malpractice suits against institutions and practitioners are commonly dismissed or withdrawn in the course of legal disputations.[15] It seems that psychiatrists are less likely than other physicians to incur malpractice claims,[16,17] and that approximately three-fourths of suits brought against psychiatrists prove unsuccessful.[18] Nevertheless, the prospects of enduring the emotional and financial demands of malpractice litigation serve as strong incentives for RM, the costs of which are usually significantly less in comparison. To reduce risk further, when harmful errors have occurred and are recognized as such, it is in the best interests of institutions and practitioners to acknowledge the errors honestly rather than trying to conceal them. Evading questions, attempting to sequester documents, and blaming others tend to alienate injured parties further and inflame their passions, while these tactics simultaneously alert litigants' lawyers to the smell of something rotten.

Institutional managerial and administrative concerns

In addition to risk matters pertaining to the care of individual patients addressed in a later section, institutional administrative responsibilities can include the following: compliance with building fire and safety codes (accompanied by periodic safety drills); maintenance of working facilities (eg, stairs, elevators, beds, and sprinklers); creation of facility evacuation plans/disaster arrangements; ensuring safe physical transfer of patients; designing secure charting and (electronic) transfer systems for communication of confidential patient information; screening, credentialing, appointment, and supervision of medical (and other) staff; ongoing evaluation of personnel and programs; ensuring stability of behavioral care institutions; and awareness of changes in political, economic, and legal climates. These responsibilities, and the risk climates surrounding them, were not always so fraught. For the bulk of the twentieth century, institutions were largely immune to suit for actions believed malfeasant. The tide turned in the 1970s in response to changes in the national mood, increased assertiveness on the part of aggrieved patients, alert attorneys, and responsive courts, and the growth in size and wealth of health care institutional providers. The number of malpractice suits consequently increased exponentially, followed in kind by increased malpractice premiums.[19] These developments led to an increased emphasis on RM and administrative responsibility for the matters cited above, in addition to the existing traditional clinical management responsibilities that include cognizance of staff approaches to assessment, diagnosis, and treatment, the nature and means of intra-staff information exchange, and the establishment of hierarchies of supervisory responsibility.

Children and RM

Children develop and pass through stages of cognitive, language, physical, and emotional maturation. Independent of stage, they are viewed legally as minors who have not attained adult status. RM comes into play with regard to guardian rights (eg, ownership of patient chart material; access to information concerning dangerous-ness; consent for care; demands for physical access to minor patients). Designation of who is the "patient" (eg, the minor or the family), shades of gray regarding confiden-tiality, lack of definition of "assent" for care, responsibility for patient safety, paucity of evidence-based data for medical decisions, conflicts in apportioning decisional responsibility, myriad definitions of "child psychotherapy," off-label or formally unap-proved uses of medications, and potential self- or other-directed dangerousness, are all areas or situations that entail risky decision-making by clinicians and therefore require knowledge of risk assessment and management.[20]

Communication and documentation

Independent of the RM matter under consideration, 2 salient principles hold: the need for clear communication between and among individuals (administrators, clinicians, and patients) and solid documentation of data, thought processes, and events. The higher the risk, the greater the need for both. Thus, the importance of a good thera-peutic alliance (itself a consequence of thorough and pleasant communication) between physician and patient is underscored. Clear communication about and understanding of individual responsibilities in the supervisory hierarchy, with docu-mented delegations of authority and role definitions, is similarly highlighted. When communication problems arise, as they inevitably do, they too should be documented, as should the ensuing follow-up and resolutions of the difficulties.

ETHICS AND RM APPLIED TO CAP

When considering ethical reasoning and RM practices applied to CAP, for heuristic purposes the focus first centers on the concerns of the CAP administrator of organi-zational units and subsequently on those of individual CAP clinicians. Although the particulars of the matters under scrutiny may differ, the approaches often overlap considerably.

Administration of Organizational Units

Several items of concern to CAP administrators, whether their units are small inpatient wards, large departments or divisions, or behavioral health organizations, are chosen for purposes of illustration.[21]

Budgeting

Budgeting for service provision invariably involves choices between the funding of certain entities at the expense of others, as the monies available for disbursement typi-cally are limited. For example, the CAP administrator choosing between funding of a new inpatient unit versus expansion of an existing outpatient service that is inadequate to meet the workload must consider which patient needs will be met and which will not. Financial considerations include total costs of the different operations, the potential payer mixes, likelihoods of ultimate profit and loss, and the degrees to which school systems and social service agencies contribute to the costs and provide services.[22] Before these commercial considerations, however, thought must be given to the target patient population's degree of need for these services and availability of professional staff: in other words, which choice is likely to benefit more patients (beneficence) and would hurt fewer (nonmalificence). Such ethical thinking implicitly engages the principle of (distributive) justice (ie, aiding the common good by providing for the largest number). RM practices also play a role: has the institution been mandated to provide services to the most acutely and severely ill (ie, emergency and inpatient care) or are other local institutions designated for that purpose? The institution with a legal obligation to provide these services but not doing so might rapidly find itself in legal jeopardy, whether actions were initiated by aggrieved patients or governmental bodies. Similarly, as inpatient and outpatient services require staff with differing specialized skills, planning for staff personnel to receive the training necessary to help particular types of patients would reduce risks resulting from inadequate delivery of care.

In the context of budgetary concerns, administrative CAP practitioners may encounter ethical conflicts and external pressures when they are faced with the choice of attending to and advocating for the needs of individuals against those of large populations of patients, to both of which they have fiduciary and legal responsibilities.[23] In such cases, the American Medical Association and American Psychiatric Association have clearly articulated that the needs of the individual patient have priority. Thus, it is expected of administrative CAPs that they will provide individual patients with information regarding the full range of treatment options, refer patients for alternative care unavailable through their business component, and provide comprehensive treatment commensurate with individual patients' needs.[24]

Credentialing, privileging, and the supervisory process

Ethics and RM considerations underlie credentialing, privileging, and supervisory processes. For example, brief interviews with staff applicants, coupled with cursory reviews of their curricula vitae, could lead to bad patient outcomes, whereas more painstaking investigation should provide greater knowledge of the individuals and bases for sounder judgments about staff appointments. Approval for the performance of medical procedures for barely qualified personnel (eg, for a child and adolescent psychiatrist to "cover" a geriatric ward on weekends) could jeopardize patient care. The driving forces supporting credentialing and appointment procedures should be the ethical concerns for patients' welfare and sparing them from harm. In turn, when shoddy investigative procedures are applied, servicing institutions and their administrators are put at greater legal and financial risk.

Supervisory process is a related concern, as ostensibly clear lines of authority may become blurred. The CAP administrator has obligations to delineate policies and procedures for staff that should include role definitions and assignations of decisional responsibility. For example, a telephoned "quiet room order" on a child psychiatric inpatient unit might not be legally acceptable unless approved by a CAP administrator. That administrator could mandate signature of such orders within a specified time period. These orders need continuous review within designated time periods, as would orders to nursing staff mandating close monitoring of the child "assigned to seclusion." These compulsory actions revolve around infringements of the children's autonomy. Their purpose, however, is to promote the child's best interests, to avoid injury, and to protect the patient, other patients, and staff. Mistakes in these procedures can lead to immediate and long-term risks for all involved parties. If, because of miscommunications or uncertainties concerning individual staff responsibilities, the patient is not given the acute care he or she requires and the patient consequently suffers, finger-pointing commonly results, which can lead to further worsening of care. When documentation of procedures, training for emergencies, and defined lines of supervisory responsibility are inadequate, the CAP administrator with ultimate responsibility for the unit will have placed patients, staff, and the institution at risk.

Documentation

Consider the following case of a troubled pediatrician. In a children's hospital, on a general medical unit, 2 adolescents, each hospitalized for several days and then discharged, engaged once in consensual unprotected sexual intercourse during their stay. The boy, who is positive for the human immunodeficiency virus (HIV), informed the pediatric attending of the incident on the day following the activity. Feeling frightened and uncertain, the attending did not chart the information. Several days later, however, the pediatrician discussed the matter with a child and adolescent psychiatrist consulting to the unit, asking for comments and advice. The attending, not the psychiatrist, has administrative responsibility for the unit, but theirs is and has been a long-term collaborative relationship, lending an appearance of authority and responsibility to the psychiatrist.

Ethical considerations and RM practices play major roles in the following analysis, which include these facts: the girl is potentially and unknowingly at risk for developing a dangerous and life-threatening illness; the boy provided the information on the assumption that it was confidential. Conflicting ethical principles are operating: the boy's autonomy rights to confidentiality versus the girl's right not to be harmed (nonmaleficence). An examination of conflicting laws between states, regarding the permissibility of conveying information about HIV status of an individual without their permission, might be factored into the considerations, although the law of any particular state should in no way dictate the outcome of an ethical analysis. That the pediatric attending was unnerved by the incident when first informed, and that out of embarrassment the facts remained undocumented, does not affect the ethical analysis. The outcome centers on granting priority either to the girl's right to be spared harm or the boy's right to confidentiality. When ethical principles profoundly conflict, it is best to choose a course of action based on the least damaging resolution.

The RM doctrines that emphasize the need for timely, comprehensive documentation and the benefits of transparency stand here in bold relief. Thus, the psychiatrist sagely advises the attending to inform his superiors and ultimately the hospital's RM and legal affairs team of the situation. These actions should in turn result in risk-reduction implementation via chart documentation of the entire matter ("better late than never"), with all relevant information transmitted to every one of the parties involved in the drama. Although doing so might result in some embarrassment for the protagonists, necessary and possibly life-saving care can then be provided, hospital procedures intended to safeguard everyone's interests would be adhered to and perhaps improved, and hospital administrative and clinical personnel (including the consulting child and adolescent psychiatrist) can operate subsequently from the relative position of strength transparency provides.

CAP research and institutional review board approvals

Primary CAP research investigators have numerous administrative factors to consider in the course of their work. Planning the focus of inquiry, inclusion and exclusion criteria for research subjects, obtaining assent and consent respectively from children and their guardians, safeguarding the rights to health and confidentiality of the participant children, arranging for the administration of protocols, collection of data and data analysis, and dissemination of findings are some of the components. Institutions and agencies commonly appoint institutional review boards (IRBs), whose purpose is to ensure that these and additional factors are sensibly addressed in study proposals.

Several ethical concerns exist in the context of children and research. Given cognitive immaturities, children are deemed incapable of fully understanding their roles in studies and consent for their participation can be given only by guardians. The effects of novel treatments on developing brains, pharmaceutical or otherwise, are largely unknown. Research studies can expose children to different degrees of risk against which the potential benefits of the outcomes have to be weighed. Federal and national organizations have focused on research ethics and their relation to children in particular,[25–27] resulting in the creation of specific ethical guidelines. Good RM practice requires adherence to these guidelines, accurate provision of the information desired by IRBs, and following the approved study protocols. Furthermore, good RM requires paying attention to appearances. Several general and CAP researchers recently experienced criticism, and their work closer scrutiny and skepticism, for alleged offenses that include expanded and inadequately validated definitions of psychiatric diagnoses, lack of transparency consequent to not publishing negative study outcomes, unreported income derived from investigative and related efforts, and encouragement of "off-label" use of psychotropic medications.[28–30] Independent of the degree of validity applicable to these allegations, the result has been the raising of questions and suspicions about the reliability and substance of a large body of work that could enhance the field's development and knowledge base. The implementation of the RM principle of transparency, and an emphasis on quality assessment to define psychiatric syndromes more rigorously and carefully prescribe psychotropic medications, are to the advantage of those child and adolescent psychiatrists administering and leading research efforts and to the specialty of CAP as a whole.

INDIVIDUAL CLINICIAN ADMINISTRATION AND PRACTICE

CAP clinicians daily engage in ethical thinking and RM practices, although they may not be aware of doing so. The clinical areas discussed and illustrated in the next section are used to heighten awareness of thoughts that commonly lurk below consciousness.

Boundaries

The individual practitioner's primary and overarching ethical responsibilities include promotion of child patients' best interests, handling those interests with integrity, being and remaining available to the children and their families as needed (fidelity), and ensuring that children are not exploited for the practitioner's benefit. The 2009 American Academy of Child and Adolescent Psychiatry (AACAP) Code of Ethics[31] expresses these sentiments, elaborates on them, and specifically addresses the matter of boundaries. Professional boundaries are imaginary separation walls, erected between physicians and patients, which foster the behaviors expected by patients and their families of their doctors, thus promoting patient safety.[32] Physicians commonly are viewed by patients as authority figures, all the more so by children who might feel powerless to protest a physician's untoward or improper breach of their autonomy or person.[33] The AACAP Code's guidelines alert child and adolescent psychiatrists to ways in which such authority can be misused, ranging from, for example, ill-advised enticements, peremptory or disrespectful handling of verbal disagreements, demanding funds from "obligated" families of patients, or most egregiously, engaging in romantic or sexual relationships with patients or family members. All of these behaviors are maleficent, that is, harmful. RM practices in these cases are simple: an awareness of proscribed behaviors, subsumed in RM terminology under risk identification and assessment, followed by the avoidance of engaging in them. To that end, child and adolescent psychiatrists are strongly advised to seek peer consultation when finding themselves in clinical situations that engender personal unease or raise ethical uncertainties.

Conflicts of Interest

As figures of authority and possessors of specialized knowledge, child and adolescent psychiatrists are positioned to influence patients' thought processes and authorize treatment approaches. Many other entities are aware of physicians' significant influence and seek to turn the child and adolescent psychiatrists' clout to their economic advantage.[34,35] As physicians who treat emotionally disturbed young people, child and adolescent psychiatrists often prescribe psychotropic medications. To remain in business and grow, pharmaceutical companies must sell their products. They need physicians to prescribe them. Ergo pharmaceutical industry advertising, promotional gifts and trinkets, offers of free lunches and dinners, stipends to "opinion leaders," sponsorship of educational seminars, and provision of medication samples.[36,37] "Big Pharma" serves as an obvious source of third-party influence. Patients' guardians, hospitals, health insurance providers, school systems, and other governmental agencies also have their self-interests and goals, prompting their attempts to influence the child and adolescent psychiatrists' clinical decisions.

The choices of one medication over another, use of a single medication versus polypharmacy, imparting confidential information about a child to a parent, timing discharge from a unit, and making recommendations about special education services to a school are all situations in which other parties, in addition to the child, have a stake. When these parties, subtly or overtly, try to influence the child and adolescent psychiatrist's decisions, by enticing for the clinician to see things their way, the clinician may face a conflict of interest. The child and adolescent psychiatrist is ethically beholden to do what is best for the patient, and must attempt to ignore seductive blandishments and avoid possible sanctions. Further, the justice principle enjoins that any one child found in a specific clinical situation will be provided with treatment equivalent to that of another child in that condition. RM considerations include reflections on the negative consequences for the child and adolescent psychiatrist that could ensue should poor clinical choices result in poor outcomes. Assigning responsibility for such choices to the alleged influences of third parties would likely prove unsuccessful as a legal defense. Identification and assessment of the risks of acceding to third-party influence or to internal motivators that do not make the child's interests primary, for example, negative countertransference toward a child or promotion of the clinician's stature, should lead directly to strategies designed to avoid or manage risks.

Assessment and Treatment

Conflicts of interest and boundary transgressions stem from child and adolescent psychiatrists paying primary attention to their needs or desires rather than, or at the expense of, those of their patients. Ethical considerations and RM awareness also play roles in those clinical situations where the needs of the patient are seen as primary, but those needs may not be adequately recognized or are mishandled, as discussed later.

Proper psychiatric care requires sufficient time for the performance of diagnostic assessments that lead to provisional diagnoses on which treatment recommendations can be based. Objections to this medical model process, centered in the past on skepticism regarding the validity of psychiatric diagnoses[38] and, separately, associated stigma,[39,40] have justifiably dwindled. However, questions concerning the current diagnostic nomenclature remain, which helps further development of the field via improved diagnostic accuracy. This stipulation regarding the necessity of the assessment process benefits child patients. Although clinicians may disagree about the validity of specific diagnoses, their applicability in a given case, and the degree of severity of a child's condition, this professional approach to cases is expected clinical behavior. Deviation from the approach immediately engenders risk for the patient and clinician, as the patient would obtain harmful care and the practitioner would face a justifiable accusation of having been responsible for it.

Once working diagnoses are established, treatments tailored to these diagnoses are in order. Although CAP seeks to develop a solid evidence base for its treatment interventions, highly specific and tailored approaches are small in number, except for emergency situations.[41,42] This is in part because most clinical cases do not involve "pure" disease manifestations but, rather, multiple confounding variables are present. Several truisms hold, nevertheless. The ability to distinguish between patients' needs for inpatient in contrast to outpatient care, knowledge of classes of medications suitable for specific psychiatric conditions, awareness of the variety of psychotherapeutic modalities and indications for their use, and cognizance of additional medical and other investigative instruments are appropriately expected of all CAP practitioners. Such practice and knowledge benefit the patient and his or her family and implicitly minimize risks for all. It is also of great help, and further minimizes risk, when the child and adolescent psychiatrist describes the course of the diagnostic process in clear terms, defines the applied diagnoses, and lays out the reasoning behind the chosen treatment recommendations. Furthermore, families often appreciate the provision of a risk/benefit analysis regarding expected outcomes in the event that recommended treatments would be pursued or declined.

Consent, Assent and Refusal of Care

Children, defined as individuals younger than 18 years, are considered to have attained cognitive and emotional maturity, from the legal perspective, on reaching that age. Independent of the accuracy of that conceptualization for a particular individual, for purposes of the law, minors (ie, youths <18 years), have limited or no legal capacity and thus are largely unable to give legal consent. Therefore, for medical care to be provided in settings other than those involving emergencies, consent must be given by the child's legal guardian. The child might or might not assent (a term that has no strict legal definition but implies voluntary agreement) to the procedure. If guardian and child agree, treatment can ensue. Should the guardian be desirous of care but the child refuse, the clinician must decide whether or not to proceed based on the degrees of objective need for care, cognitive capacities of the child, and rationales for refusal. For example, a 9-year-old child who is having a tantrum and has been diagnosed with recent onset of a specific phobia (eg, school avoidance/refusal) might require rapid intervention despite her lack of assent; by contrast, a clinician would be wise to not put a 16-year-old girl in the patient role, against her will, when the parent's chief complaint concerns a drop in the child's grades from "straight As" to "Bs." (Parenthetically, provision of advice or counseling to the parent may work as well or better.) Despite the child and adolescent psychiatrist's interest in providing benefit to the child, autonomy must be respected, and violations of autonomy rights could be harmful to the child's well-being. Beyond these ethical concerns, risk reduction occurs, independent of the decisions a child and adolescent psychiatrist might make concerning initiation of care, when the clinician's reasoning is clearly documented and verbally transmitted to the family. The latter action subsumes the concepts of informed consent and assent. Furthermore, by attending to the child's desires for or antagonisms to treatment, the clinician clearly indicates an interest in avoiding multiple agentry. Thus, the clinician's stance would not represent the interests or desires of the guardians; rather, the child and adolescent psychiatrist would be acting as an advocate for the child and his or her best interests.

Dangerousness and Confidentiality

Maintenance of children's safety is the most prominent clinical consideration. Not uncommonly, situations arise in which a child's safety is open to question. Should the child declare, verbally or by action, his or her intention to harm self or others, regard for the child's autonomy rights must be compromised while protections are arranged, possibly against his or her will, for the child and potential victims. The child's rights to confidentiality of verbal expression are breached, as the remarks are used by clinicians to prevent self-harm and warn intended victims. The duties to not cause harm or aid its occurrence (nonmaleficence) serve as the ethical underpinnings. The "duty to act," and the risks attendant to not doing so, serve as legal underpinnings.[43] Some clinical situations, however, suggest or hint at dangers rather than being overt manifestations; others may be overt but not imminent; and in still other circumstances "dangerousness" is perceived as a significant presence by some clinicians although not by their peers. For example, the youth who rides his motorbike on streets that are used by automobiles and enjoys the risk; the boy who claims to have the potential to enter, in undetectable fashion, his school's computer system and alter grades on student transcripts; the girl who engages in unprotected sexual activity, and denies such behavior to her curious and anxious parent; or the girl who sneaks occasional swigs of alcohol from the parental bar, where her parents keep their marijuana stash. In the guise of "doing good" for the patient, some clinicians might feel tempted to intervene in any or all of these scenarios by breaching their patient's confidentiality rights and informing the guardians. Likely outcomes could include engendering patients' long-term distrust of mental health personnel and refusals to participate in further treatments.

CAP clinicians also shoulder ethical responsibilities when considering discharge from hospitals of patients previously thought or adjudged "dangerous." The child and adolescent psychiatrist must feel confident that the child will not be in imminent danger post discharge, and must also make reasonable arrangements for subsequent care. The psychiatrist may also have to act as advocate (fidelity principle) for the child in the event of disagreement with caretaking guardians. For example, the psychiatrist could conclude, based on safety concerns, that hospitalization of a youngster is necessary, although the guardians find such a decision disagreeable or inconvenient. Good RM practice demands clear documentation and communication of the reasons behind the choice to reduce discomfort and promote accommodation to the treatment plan.

Issues around confidentiality rights often arise for clinicians, most commonly in the context of communications with adolescents. When the possible need for disclosure of private information is identified, the clinician will inevitably feel squeezed. A preferred management strategy is to approach such cases from the outset with a family perspective rather than concentrating the focus on the adolescent. Thus, it would initially be made explicit that all family member communications are considered potentially conveyable by the child and adolescent psychiatrist to others. Furthermore, all parties would be informed that this action would definitely be exercised in the event of "dangerousness," although the psychiatrist's judgment and tact would govern handling of other individual communications.

Confidentiality concerns for child and adolescent psychiatrists also arise in connection with matters of documentation and transmission of information. Guardians legally have access to their children's chart notes. Problems can arise when, for example, parents seek documentation to obtain governmental or insurance benefits for their children; divorcing parents engage in custody fights; other professionals, schools, courts, or agencies request or require information concerning children they serve. Good RM practice requires judicious management of such requests. Chart documentation should be limited to the factual and gratuitous remarks avoided, with the comments of other caretakers and intimates noted as quotes with attribution. Confidential information should be conveyed only in the event of a guardian's signed consent and, ideally, with the assent of the child. Guardians and the child patient should know the specific information that is to be conveyed. Information sufficient to answer specific questions should be submitted, rather than entire patient records. Recently established federal Health Insurance Portability and Accountability Act (HIPAA) regulations[44] governing transmission of personal medical information (increasingly often at the touch of a keyboard key) contains safeguards against its inappropriate use, but these protections are not foolproof and ownership of child-related information can become murky.[45] Thus, awareness and use of all these risk-avoidance practices is important to the responsible handling of patient records.

SUMMARY

Ethical thinking and RM practices are frequent bedfellows, although, as illustrated in this article, they derive from different concerns and sources. This article has reviewed several traditional categories of ethical concerns, such as confidentiality, boundaries, and assent/consent, and RM concerns centered on, for example, dangerousness, credentialing, and information transfer. The use of the invaluable ethical reasoning process, and the needs for good documentation practices and interpersonal and interstaff communication in these arenas, cannot be overemphasized. These approaches are crucial to the practice of good administrative CAP, be it the management of staff, institutional units, or agencies, or the administrative aspects of treating individual patients by individual practitioners.

In addition to traditional ethical and RM concerns, it is important to anticipate future developments touching on these areas. For example, given the ease of globalized electronic access available to huge numbers of people, might the ethically based view of the confidentiality of medical records rapidly become a quaint and passé notion? Similarly, given the ease of access to medical information available to the public on the Internet, might physicians be more readily accused of providing inadequate care, in turn causing harm, if their care suggests a lack of awareness of new developments in their fields? Furthermore, the advent of genomics and genetically based individualized care could become the expected standard of care, rendering current approaches ethically inadequate and risky. At present, the relationships between practitioners and the pharmaceutical industry are undergoing significant upheavals. These changes, resulting from ethical conflict of interest concerns and possibly risky clinical practices, are likely to affect future practice patterns, availability of research monies, and provisions of medical knowledge and education. As change and development continue inexorably, in medical mores as in children, ethical and RM challenges will similarly continue to evolve and administrative approaches will have to adapt, in the enduring effort to provide beneficial, nonharmful care while simultaneously reducing the risk exposure of CAP managers and practitioners.

REFERENCES

1. Martin A, Volkmar F, editors. Lewis's child and adolescent psychiatry: a comprehensive textbook. Philadelphia: Wolters Kluwer; 2007.
2. Bloch S, Green S. The scope of psychiatric ethics. In: Bloch S, Green S, editors. Psychiatric ethics. 4th edition. Oxford (UK): Oxford University Press; 2009. p. 3–8.
3. Beauchamp T, Childress J. Principles of biomedical ethics. 6th edition. Oxford (UK): Oxford University Press; 2008.
4. Crouhy M, Galai D, Mark R. The essentials of risk management. New York: McGraw-Hill; 2006.
5. Carroll R, American Society for Healthcare Risk Management. Risk management handbook for health care organizations. San Francisco (CA): Jossey-Bass; 2001.
6. Bloch S. Care ethics: what psychiatrists have been waiting for to make sound ethical decisions. Psychiatr Ann 2007;37:787–91.
7. Sondheimer A, Jensen P. Ethics and child and adolescent psychiatry. In: Bloch S, Green S, editors. Psychiatric ethics. 4th edition. Oxford (UK): Oxford University Press; 2009. p. 385–407.
8. Childress J. The normative principles of medical ethics. In: Veatch R, editor. Medical ethics. 2nd edition. Boston: Jones and Bartlett; 1997.
9. Jonsen A, Siegler M, Winslade W. Clinical ethics: a practical approach to ethical decisions in clinical medicine. New York: McGraw-Hill; 2002.
10. Available at: http://en.wikipedia.org/wiki/risk_management. Accessed January 7, 2009.
11. Schetky D. Medical errors: my three perspectives. AACAP. Acad News 2008;39: 276–7.
12. Dorfman M. Introduction to risk management and insurance. 9th edition. Englewood Cliffs (NJ): Prentice Hall; 2007.
13. Simon R, Shuman D. Clinical manual of psychiatry and law. Arlington (VA): American Psychiatric Publications; 2007.
14. Flach F. A comprehensive guide to malpractice risk management in psychiatry. New York: Hatherleigh Press; 1998.
15. Tsao C, Layde J. A basic review of psychiatric medical malpractice law in the United States. Compr Psychiatry 2007;48:309–12.
16. Slawson P. Psychiatric malpractice: the low frequency risks. Med Law 1993;12: 673–80.
17. Morrison J, Morrison T. Psychiatrists disciplined by a state medical board. Am J Psychiatry 2001;158:474–8.
18. Simon R. Clinical-legal issues in psychiatry. In: Sadock B, Sadock V, editors. Comprehensive textbook of psychiatry. 8th edition. Philadelphia: Lippincott Williams & Wilkins; 2005. p. 3969–88.
19. Richards. E III. The professional liability insurance crisis. Available at: http://biotech.law.lsu.edu/Books/aspen-The-4.html. Accessed January 7, 2009.
20. The Psychiatrists' Program. Risk management issues in the psychiatric treatment of children and adolescents. Available at: http://www.psychprogram.com/FPO/library/rm-0133.aspx. Accessed December 23, 2008.

21. Medical Risk Management. preventive legal strategies for health care providers – contents. Available at: http://biotech.law.lsu.edu/Books/aspen/Aspen-Contents.html. Accessed January 7, 2009.

22. Villani S. Children's services. In: Talbott J, Hales R, editors. Textbook of administrative psychiatry: new concepts for a changing behavioral health system. 2nd edition. Washington DC: American Psychiatric Publishing; 2001. p. 313–22.

23. Sabin J, Daniels N. Determining medical necessity in mental health practice. Hastings Cent Rep 1994;24:5–14.

24. Lazarus J. Ethics. In: Talbott J, Hales R, editors. Textbook of administrative psychiatry: new concepts for a changing behavioral health system. 2nd edition. Washington DC: American Psychiatric Publishing; 2001. p. 379–85.

25. National Commission for the Protection of Human Subjects of Biomedical and Behavioral Research. Research involving children: report and recommendations. Washington DC: DHEW Publication No. (OS) 77–0005; 1977.

26. Department of Health and Human Services. Protection of human subjects: research involving children. Fed Regist 1983;48:9814–20.

27. Department of Health and Human Services. OPRR Reports: protection of human subjects. Fed Regist 1991;46:115–408.

28. Harris G, Carey B. Researchers fail to reveal full drug pay. New York Times. June 8, 2008; A1.

29. Harris G, Carey B, Roberts J. Psychiatrists, troubled children, and drug industry's role. New York Times. May 10, 2007; A1, A24.

30. Fontanarosa P, Flanagin A, DeAngelis C. Reporting conflicts of interests, financial aspects of research, and role of sponsors in funded studies. JAMA 2005;294: 110–1.

31. American Academy of Child and Adolescent Psychiatry. Code of ethics. Available at: http://www.AACAP.org/galleries/AboutUs/CodeofEthics.pdf. Accessed February 22, 2009.

32. Gutheil T, Gabbard G. The concept of boundaries in clinical practice: theoretical and risk-management dimensions. Am J Psychiatry 1993;150:188–96.

33. Schetky D. Boundaries in child and adolescent psychiatry. In: Schetky D, editor. Child and adolescent psychiatric clinics of North America. Philadelphia: Saunders; 1995. p. 769–78.

34. Lewis D, Michels R, Pine D, et al. Conflict of interest. Am J Psychiatry 2006;163: 571–3.

35. Cain D, Detsky A. Everyone's a little bit biased (even physicians). JAMA 2008; 299:2893–5.

36. Wazana A, Primeau F. Ethical considerations in the relationship between physicians and the pharmaceutical industry. Psychiatr Clin North Am 2002; 25:647–63.

37. Campbell E. Doctors and drug companies – scrutinizing influential relationships. N Engl J Med 2007;357:1796–7.

38. Pies R. How "objective" are psychiatric diagnoses? Psychiatry 2007;4:18–22.

39. Pescosolido B, Perry B, Martin J, et al. Stigmatizing attitudes and beliefs about treatment and psychiatric medications for children with mental illness. Psychiatr Serv 2007;58:613–8.

40. Rosen A, Walter G, Casey D, et al. Combating psychiatric stigma: an overview of contemporary initiatives. Australas Psychiatry 2000;8:19–26.

41. McClellan J, Werry J. Evidence-based treatments in child and adolescent psychiatry. J Am Acad Child Adolesc Psychiatry 2003;42:1388–400.

42. Kazdin A, Weisz J. Evidence-based psychotherapies for children and adolescents. New York: Guilford; 2003.

43. Kachigian C, Felthous A. Court responses to Tarasoff statutes. J Am Acad Psychiatry Law 2004;32:263–73.

44. Department of Health and Human Services. Standards for Privacy of Individually Identifiable Health Information (the Privacy Rule), 45 CFR Parts 160 and 164 (adopted April, 2001).

45. Alessi N. Information technology and child and adolescent psychiatry. Behav Health Trends 2001;13:24–9.

Advocating for Children and Adolescents with Mental Illnesses

Kristin Kroeger Ptakowski, BA

KEYWORDS

- Policy • Congress • Legislation • Advocacy
- Mental health parity

The mental health community has made tremendous strides over the last 20 years to eradicate stigma, demand policy change, and improve the lives of millions of children and adolescents with mental illnesses. Most of this has been accomplished through advocacy at all levels of government and was assisted by community involvement. However, addressing access to care for children and adolescents with mental illnesses is still a challenge. Despite 2 decades of dedicated effort, there remain many children and adolescents with mental illness without health insurance. Workforce shortages in child psychiatrists,[1] inadequate reimbursement of health care costs, limited government-supported research funding, and lack of coordinated systems of care result in persistent barriers to effective mental health care. Emergency rooms are still often the only resort for treatment. Building on past successes and working toward improvements within child mental health systems can be done by better informing our policy makers about needs and deficiencies in access to care and by urging our legislators to improve the lives of millions of children and adolescent with mental illnesses.

Advocacy is a challenging concept because there is no one set of instructions about where and how to begin and what constitutes effectiveness. Advocacy can mean many things, but fundamentally, it is about speaking out and making a case for something important and about supporting a cause. It can be political, as in lobbying for a specific piece of legislation, or social, as in speaking out on behalf of those without a voice. Legislators and their staff in our federal and state governments are often unaware of children's mental health issues. Child and adolescent psychiatrists may be instrumental in drafting, debating, and implementing the laws and regulations that govern child and adolescent mental health care, individually or together with

American Academy of Child and Adolescent Psychiatry, 3615 Wisconsin Avenue NW, Washington, DC 20016, USA
E-mail address: kkroeger@aacap.org

Child Adolesc Psychiatric Clin N Am 19 (2010) 131–138
doi:10.1016/j.chc.2009.08.003
1056-4993/09/$ – see front matter © 2010 Elsevier Inc. All rights reserved.

organizations dedicated to the needs of children and families. Elected officials look to professionals for advice or recommendations for developing policy initiatives because their voice is one of authority and expertise in child and adolescent mental health.

The reasons for advocacy need to be explored. Fortunately, when more people get involved, wonderful things can happen. All the legislative victories of recent decades—educational rights for children with disabilities, state and federal mental health parity, environmental protection, child care for working parents—are the direct result of advocacy. Getting involved in advocacy will not always yield success, but being uninvolved never does so. People may think that they do not have time, may not know where to start, or may be intimidated, but advocacy can also be enjoyable. Advocacy includes working directly with legislators and policy makers, working with a school administration to meet the unique needs of the child, appealing against denial of specific treatment or formulary approval by the managed care company, and educating and collaborating with primary care physicians on appropriate treatments.

Three principles that need to be understood about advocating are that change takes time, persistence is absolute, and compromise is inevitable.

A new Congress begins every 2 years and new state assemblies typically begin each year. Each new legislature brings new faces and priorities, making reintroduction of bills a necessity. Showing persistence, building on what has been developed previously, and moving forward are important. The way to advance an agenda is often grounded in compromise and in the ability to create a strategy for future initiatives.

CHANGE TAKES TIME

Mental health policy issues are far from new; in fact, many issues have roots that go back 50 years or more. In health policy, as in other areas of policymaking, history has played out in often unexpected ways. In the early 1950s, it was unheard of to educate children with mental illness in the classroom. Throughout the late 1950s and 60s, laws, such as the Training of Professional Personnel Act of 1959 (public law [PL] 86–158), were enacted to help train leaders to educate children with intellectual disabilities. The Elementary and Secondary Education Act (PL 89–10) and the State Schools Act (PL 89–313) provided states with direct grant assistance to help educate children with disabilities. Finally, the Handicapped Children's Early Education Assistance Act of 1968 (PL 90–538) authorized support for exemplary early childhood programs and increased Head Start enrollment for young children with disabilities.[2] These and other critical federal laws paved the way for Congress to enact the Education for All Handicapped Children Act (PL 94–142) in 1975 (now called the Individuals with Disabilities Act), which began opening up educational opportunity for children with disabilities and their families.

In 1983, with a Congressional mandate and funding, the National Institute of Mental Health initiated the Child and Adolescent Service System Program. This program provided funds and technical assistance to the states and territories to plan and develop systems of care for children with serious emotional disturbance. In 1986, Congress passed the State Comprehensive Mental Health Services Plan Act that required all states to develop and implement plans to create community-based service systems for all persons with mental illnesses. Building on these successes, in 1992, Congress created and funded the Comprehensive Community Mental Health Services for Children and their Families Program; today, this program is the major source of funding for local systems of care development.

It is clear from this brief history that effective policy change takes time and its foundation is often rooted in other successful legislative initiatives.

PERSISTENCE IS ABSOLUTE

Time, patience, and perseverance will accomplish all things.
–Anonymous.

Advocacy can include activities like organizing a community march, writing a letter to the editor, testifying before your county board, or writing to or visiting one's elected officials. The most basic form of advocacy is just "speaking up." However, many will listen but not hear the message the first time, and continuing to speak up about the issue is vital to successful advocacy.

Clarity, brevity, and use of language that everyone understands, including those that are not experts on the specific issues, is important. Every communication, in person, by phone, or in writing, should have one basic message, for example, "There is a severe shortage of child and adolescent psychiatrists and this is how we can resolve it. . ." One should not be afraid to repeat this message until the right person listens.

COMPROMISE IS INEVITABLE: THE 80% RULE

There is tremendous exhilaration in "winning," but there is also a lot of satisfaction in just advancing a mission. When advocating at the local, state, or federal level, change takes time. Often, only part of the requested change will happen, but with the right strategies, it can be a step and sometimes a leap forward.

Very few pieces of legislation are passed with 100% of what any one constituency wants. Wyoming Senator Mike Enzi said that he hoped to help overcome partisanship in Congress with his "80 percent rule"—his belief that Democrats and Republicans can get more done by focusing on the 80% on which they can agree.[3] Often constituencies advocating for a piece of legislation say that they can support most of the provisions on the table, but there is 20% that they cannot support or that may be missing. The problem for so many reformers is that some are likely to "fall on their sword" over the 20% and kill the entire piece of legislation. Advocates play a critical role in identifying the points of consensus between the constituents and recommending legislation based on compromise, rather than abandoning the potential change altogether.

The Paul Wellstone and Pete Domenici Mental Health Parity and Addiction Equity Act of 2008[4] provides an example of a successful legislative act that incorporates the 3 components of waiting for positive change, being persistent, and facing the inevitable need for compromise. From the early 1990s to 2008, small steps were made to improve the discrimination against people with mental illnesses in their health insurance coverage. In its proposal for health care reform in 1994, the Clinton administration attempted to shift the burden from the consumer to the public or private insurance sectors by introducing a mental health parity law.[5] The Clinton health reform bill never advanced but it was instrumental in a trend toward mental health parity and the redistribution of mental health care provided by health maintenance organizations. In September 1996, the Mental Health Parity Act (MHPA) of 1996 was introduced. This was the first legislation to make mental health annual or lifetime dollar limits equal to those that applied to medical or surgical benefits. After a failed attempt to amend this bill to an overall health care bill, it was attached to a Veterans and Housing Appropriations bill and passed, but only after significant compromises. In 2001 and subsequent years, legislation was enacted to expand the 1996 mental health parity law. Although some of the bills were passed in one chamber, the other chamber did not approve them, and thus the bills did not become law. For years, laws that extended the time period of the 1996 MHPA were the only legislative advances in mental health care.

However, between 1996 and 2007, two different constituencies, the mental health community (providers and family advocates), and the health insurance companies were discussing how they could work together to improve health insurance coverage for persons with mental illnesses. In 2008, these efforts led to the enactment of the Paul Wellstone and Pete Domenici Mental Health Parity and Addiction Equity Act. This too did not pass without compromises, such as requiring health plans to continue coverage of the disorders and treatments that they currently cover, rather than mandating that health plans provide coverage for every mental health disorder published in the diagnostic and statistical manual of mental disorders. However, through the persistence of the mental health community group, with the passage of the act, imposing different treatment or financial limitations in health plans on mental health benefits from those applied to medical and surgical services is now prohibited. The legislation successfully closed the loopholes that allow discrimination in the co-payments, coinsurance, deductibles, maximum out-of-pocket limits, and day and visit limits.

JOINING TOGETHER TO EFFECT CHANGE
Identifying Allies

Demonstrating to elected officials that one is representing many constituencies, institutions, and voters in one's community is important. To begin advocacy efforts, it is important to scan the environment for allies and opponents. For child and adolescent psychiatrists, likely allies are the families and youth being treated. Other pediatric physician colleagues, child psychologists, social workers, school counselors, and teachers can also be allies in advocacy. Discussing the issues of access to mental health care with these allies will help to illuminate how a policy might affect child and adolescent psychiatrists, families, and other professionals.

Professional organizations, such as American Academy of Child and Adolescent Psychiatry (AACAP) are also allies and resources. Professional organizations have staff to monitor policy issues, alert the membership to upcoming legislation and regulatory action, and meet with members of Congress on the organization's behalf. They can also arrange meetings with elected representative at the state and federal levels. Professional organizations often collaborate with other groups to draw on everyone's knowledge and jointly activate numerous organizations at the grassroots level. The larger the number of cooperating individuals and organizations, the more effective advocacy efforts will be.

Principles of Legislative Advocacy

Timing advocacy to influence legislation is an important skill. Once an issue is decided by vote, it is difficult, often practically impossible, to reverse the decision until the next year or the next session of Congress. As mentioned earlier, passing legislation can take a long time and just because a piece of legislation is not advancing, it does not mean that it is not supported. Other influences, such as policy cost, political wrangling, or competing priorities, can hold up a piece of legislation. The shortage of children's mental health professionals has been a priority of the AACAP for many years. Legislation called the Child Healthcare Crisis Relief Act,[6] which provides loan forgiveness and scholarships to individuals who study in graduate and medical programs in child mental health, was first introduced in 2004 and reintroduced in subsequent years. Even though the bill gained support each year and ultimately was amended to another piece of legislation, it has not been adopted. With the focus on mental health parity legislation last year, discussions about this bill were put on hold. However, the passage of the MHPA provides an opportunity to move this legislation forward using the argument that with equal insurance coverage, more individuals will be seeking mental health care; consequently, the shortage of children's mental health professionals is a real concern and an impediment to treatment access.

Once policy is introduced, it is important to consult allies and decide on a strategy. There are 100 members of the US Senate and 438 members of the House of Representatives, including the delegates from the District of Columbia and the US territories, which makes the task of educating them about a specific policy issue daunting. A targeted approach is paramount to making the best use of resources.

Firstly, it is important to decide which elected representatives might be "champions" for the legislation. Getting bipartisan support is essential. The mental health community has wonderful champions in Representative Patrick Kennedy, former Representative Jim Ramstad, Senator Edward Kennedy, and former Senator Pete Domenici. All have shown a commitment to improving the lives of children and adolescents with mental illness. Secondly, it is important to know which committees and subcommittees have jurisdiction over the legislation. If legislation is introduced and referred to a committee, this does not mean that the committee will discuss it. It is up to advocates to inform policy makers about its importance and garner support.

Once the champions are recognized and strategies are set, there are various ways to communicate the message. Avenues for communicating with public offices include:

- Visiting, telephoning, writing, or sending a fax or e-mail to the congressional district or Washington, DC office
- Attending rallies, fundraisers, or town hall meetings where the champions are expected to speak
- Inviting elected officials to a local child psychiatry meeting, hospital, or clinic
- Writing a letter to the editor for placement in a local or state paper and taking advantage of other media opportunities

Communicating with Legislators

Research has shown that almost half of all Americans had been in touch with a member of congress in the last 5 years.[7] It was in the mid-1990s that congressional offices got e-mail addresses and before that, most communication was done by mail, fax, and telephone contact. The advent of the Internet and other wireless communication continues to significantly ease becoming involved in the public policy process. The Internet and e-mail have also provided grassroots and professional organizations with new and exciting opportunities to organize around issues and to access and share information. President Barak Obama's 2008 campaign took full advantage of various technologies to create a "netroots," that mobilized voters across the country into a unified voice.[8]

Many who contact Congress are motivated and assisted in doing so by professional and advocacy organizations. These organizations provide significant guidance and assistance with the process of transmitting, and often of drafting, the communications. The AACAP provides specific language and other talking points for e-mail, fax, or telephone communication.[9]

The most effective way to quickly communicate your message to your elected official depends on the specific legislators and their staff. Although members of Congress genuinely want to hear from constituents, the rising volume of communication from them has overwhelmed their collective staff. Because congressional offices function basically as independent small businesses, each office's staff have had to decide how to manage its messages. E-mails from personal or work (if appropriate) computers are always best. Some offices have concluded that advocacy campaigns of identical form messages that are not sent from constituents' addresss or under their name do not warrant a response.[10]

E-mail and telephone is the easiest and most standard way to communicate your message, although there is no substitute for face-to-face communication with one's elected official or staff. This often cannot be done on a weekly or even monthly basis but should be done once a year. Elected representative are available for meetings in their district offices within the state or in Washington, DC. AACAP and other professional advocacy organizations can assist with making the appointments and provide material for the meeting. Congressional representatives are very busy and may not be able to meet with their constituents for long periods or at all. It is important to get to know not only elected officials but also their staff, who often do the "real," behind-the-scenes work. They are often more knowledgeable than the representative about one's issues. Congressional staff are highly valuable to their bosses and are essentially tasked with prioritizing the many request made by constituents. Interaction with the staff is often the critical link in making certain that the issues are seen by the representative.

Many professional organizations have organized days to visit elected representatives. For the last 4 years, AACAP has held an advocacy day and invited child and adolescent psychiatrists from across the country to Washington, DC to learn about the legislative process and meet with their Congressional offices. It is important to invite allies, such as families, to join the meetings. By including different viewpoints, the meeting will be seen as representing multiple constituencies. By meeting face-to-face with elected representatives or their staff, communication lines are opened and dialog can begin. Local professionals often become their experts and are sought out for advice afterwards.

Important points to remember when calling, sending e-mails, or meeting elected representatives include

- Mentioning that one is a constituent and a child and adolescent psychiatrist and mentioning one's other professional affiliations, such as affiliation to a large university, hospital, or business in that district or state
- Keeping the message simple, using language that everyone will understand, and spelling out acronyms such as GME (graduate medial education)
- Including a personal anecdote about why taking a specific action is needed; for example, when asking for support with legislation to address the shortage of children's mental health professionals, providing information on the average wait time for a new patient to be seen due to an already excessive case load

When meeting with an elected official, visual aids or charts are powerful tools to emphasize key points. One must be prepared for follow-up questions. Not knowing information that they want is acceptable, because getting back to them with it is a great way to reconnect and continue the dialog. Postmeeting contact via email or telephone is important for reinforcing the message.

Many members of Congress are in their home district or state on the weekends and also take designated recesses throughout the year. During these times, they often attend town hall meetings, state fairs, fundraisers, and other public events to talk with their constituents. These are ideal opportunities to ask questions about specific policy issues. For a more intimate acquaintance with elected officials and to educate them on specific policy concerns, invite them to a local professional organization . Presenting them with an award is another avenue for showing support.

Working with Media

The media are an extremely powerful tool for policy change. Public awareness will help build a larger constituency for one's issue and further strengthen advocacy efforts. The goal of connecting with the media is to influence behavior or policies and to offer information on problems and solutions that otherwise might be ignored.[11] Two media tools include writing a letter to the editor and developing a relationship with a local journalist, requesting that an editorial be written. Although repeating statistics on a specific topic is not media advocacy, using those statistics to push for stronger laws or enforcement of existing ones is considered so. Elected officials and their staff watch television, listen to the radio, and read their local newspapers to better understand what issues are "hot" in their area. To keep specific issues in people's minds, getting journalists' attention, understanding what they want, and making those issues newsworthy is important. No opportunity must be missed to publically acknowledge a legislator's commitment to one's issues through a letter to the editor. Too often, legislators only get recognized for mistakes; if they are supportive of one's issues, a public acknowledgment may encourage other elected officials to be aware of the issues and possibly support them.

STATE LEVEL ADVOCACY

Advocacy on the state and local level is as important as work on the federal level. Today, the relationship between the states and the federal government in shaping and implementing public policy and the connection between federal and state public policy is becoming more evident. Because of this environment, public policy advocacy is critical at the state and federal level. Many laws and regulations that have the biggest impact on our everyday lives are passed at the state and local level. When a program, such as the State Children's Health Insurance Program, is passed by Congress, it is state legislatures that decide on how it will be implemented in their state. Likewise, because the constitution relegates basic police powers to the states, policies on juvenile justice and offenders with mental health problems are written and implemented at state level.

The methods for communication with one's state officials is similar to federal officials, however, there are some differences:

- Elected and appointed officials are more approachable.
- Public testimony is often sought.
- If a bill gains momentum in one state, it is easier to pass in another.

Elected and appointed officials often live on a day-to-day basis in the community that they represent. They are more accessible and approachable and taking advantage of this is important. It is estimated that state legislatures consider over 100,000 bills a year. Many state elected officials do not have a large staff, if any at all. With the vast number of bills introduced, no legislator is an expert, and advocates for child and adolescent psychiatry can be a valuable tool.[12] Committees often hold hearings where members of the public can give brief testimony and act as expert witnesses—another avenue for one's message to be heard. If legislation catches on in one state, it is often easier for another state to pass similar legislation. This gives advocates the opportunity for faster advancement of their legislation.

SUMMARY

Anatole France said , "To accomplish great things, we must not only act, but also dream, not only plan, but also believe."

The political process is most often a marathon and rarely a sprint. Persistence is needed to advance all policy objectives. Professionals, such as child and adolescent psychiatrists, play an important role in the lives of countless youth and their families across the country. Experts in child and adolescent mental health issues have the opportunity to influence policy change at all levels of government. Becoming involved in future policy changes can yield improvements in the health care delivery systems, increase in numbers of children's mental health professionals, and increases in funding for child and adolescent mental health.

REFERENCES

1. New Freedom Commission on Mental Health. Achieving the promise: transforming mental health care in America. Final report. Rockville (MD): DHHS Pub. No. SMA-03-3832; 2003.
2. Office of Special Education Programs. U.S. department of education. history: twenty five years of progress. In: Educating children with disabilities through IDEA. Available at: http://www.ed.gov/policy/speced/leg/idea/history.html. 2007. Accessed February, 2009.
3. Wyoming Sen. Enzi announces re-election campaign, ending speculation. Associated press. April 26, 2008.
4. Pete Domenici and Paul Wellstone Mental Health Parity Act. Public Law No: 110–343 (2008).
5. Department of Health and Human Services. Mental health: a report of the surgeon general. Rockville (MD): 1999. Available at: http://www.surgeongeneral.gov/library/mentalhealth/toc.html. Accessed April 8, 2002.
6. Child healthcare crisis relief Act of 2009, HR 1932, 11th Cong, 1st session (2009). Available at: http://www.thomas.gov.
7. Goldschmidt Kathy, Ochreiter Leslie. Communicating with congress: how the internet has changed citizen engagement. Washington, DC: CMF; 2008. 10–11.
8. Libert B, Faulk R. Barack, Inc.: Upper saddle river, New Jersey Pearson Education, Inc; 2009.
9. American Academy of Child and Adolescent Psychiatry. Advocacy section. Available at: http://www.aacap.org/cs/advocacy. Accessed April 15, 2009.
10. Fitch Brad, Goldschmidt Kathy. In: Communicating with Congress: How Capitol Hill is Coping with the Surge in Citizen Advocacy, 31. Washington, DC: CMF; 2005. Available at: http://www.cmfweb.org/storage/cmfweb/documents/CMF_Pubs/communicatingwithcongress_report1.pdf. Accessed February, 2009.
11. Efroymson Debra. Using media and research for advocacy: low cost ways to increase success. HealthBridge; 2006.
12. American Academy of Child and Adolescent Psychiatry. State Government Advocacy Manual. 2007. Available at: http://www.aacap.org/galleries/stateadvocacy/2007StateGovernmentAdvocacyManual.pdf. Accessed February, 2009.

Developing Effective Child Psychiatry Collaboration with Primary Care: Leadership and Management Strategies

Barry D. Sarvet, MD[a],*, Lynn Wegner, MD, FAAP[b]

KEYWORDS

- Health services accessibility • Child psychiatry
- Primary health care • Practice management

Despite major strides in the understanding and treatment of psychiatric disorders in children during the past 2 decades, studies have shown that the vast majority of those suffering from these disorders do not receive mental health treatment.[1] Not only is there a persistent workforce shortage for child and adolescent psychiatrists (CAPs), but there is a host of formidable barriers (economic, structural barriers, stigma, cultural factors) that prevents many children and families from obtaining psychiatric care.[2] Unfortunately, traditional models of office-based child psychiatric practice, designed to deliver excellent treatment to a relatively small panel of patients, do not offer solutions to this serious problem of inadequate access to care. Those highly motivated or financially well-endowed families who manage to get into these panels, while certainly deserving of the care they receive, represent only a very small fraction of the public health burden of child psychiatric illness.

In recent years, there has been a growing interest in the idea of collaborative practice in child and adolescent psychiatry. CAPs may collaborate with systems and caregivers for children including parents, schools, community centers, religious

[a] Division of Child and Adolescent Psychiatry, Baystate Medical Center, Tufts University School of Medicine, 3300 Main Street, 4th Floor, Springfield, MA 01199, USA
[b] Division of Developmental and Behavioral Pediatrics, University of North Carolina School of Medicine, Chapel Hill, NC, USA
* Corresponding author.
E-mail address: barry.sarvet@baystatehealth.org (B.D. Sarvet).

Child Adolesc Psychiatric Clin N Am 19 (2010) 139–148
doi:10.1016/j.chc.2009.08.004
1056-4993/09/$ – see front matter © 2010 Elsevier Inc. All rights reserved.

institutions, other mental health providers, and of course, other health care providers. The collaborative child psychiatrist respects and recognizes the strengths of these systems, joins with them, and thereby brings his or her expertise into the places where children and families can be found. One of these places is the pediatrician's office.

As medical colleagues, pediatricians are natural and likely partners, but child psychiatrists and pediatricians have a complicated history together. Many pediatricians are understandably uncomfortable with their role in the treatment of mental health problems for children who "slip between the cracks" of poorly coordinated systems of mental health care.[3] Too often, their calls to child psychiatrists are unanswered, referrals ignored, and pediatric charts of patients in longstanding psychiatric care lack correspondence from the treating child psychiatrist.

Yet, pediatricians are in a unique position to serve a vital role in the prevention, early detection, initial management, and coordination of care for childhood mental illness. Although training of pediatricians in mental health and psychiatry has been considered inadequate,[4] pediatricians have long recognized the importance of mental health and psychosocial factors in the development of children. Generations of parents have received counsel from pediatricians regarding child rearing practices and behavior management. Unlike child psychiatrists, experienced general pediatricians have seen large numbers of children with healthy development, providing them with an excellent vantage point for detecting deviations in development and knowing when problems are serious. Unlike child psychiatrists, pediatricians do "checkups," also known as well-child visits, during which children are screened for early signs of disease and parents are given anticipatory guidance for the management of preclinical health problems. For example, in 2002, 86% of insured children and 71% of uninsured children younger than 6 years had a well-child visit with a health professional in the past year.[5] There is usually no stigma or shame associated with a visit to the pediatrician's office. Pediatricians are increasingly recognizing the need and opportunity for their practices to become a "medical home" for children by providing family-centered coordination of care for children with special health care needs.[6]

Through collaboration, CAPs enable the pediatrician to do so much more than respond to the dreaded "Friday afternoon crisis," and help to establish a clear place for mental health within a context of prevention and health promotion for all children. In this way, CAPs can help far more children and families than would be possible in traditional practice.

ADMINISTRATIVE AND FINANCIAL BARRIERS TO COLLABORATION

Unfortunately, it is not by accident that contemporary child psychiatrists have found it difficult to maintain collaborative relationships with primary care providers (PCPs). Mental health services seem to exist in a system apart from the general health care system, even when they occur in the same organization. This situation is represented and reinforced by separate ("carved out") insurance and payment systems, separate billing codes (Current Procedural Terminology [CPT] Psychiatry and Psychology Specialty codes[7]), separate medical record systems and practices, and separate state regulatory systems. Reimbursement for the substantial indirect time and effort required to bridge the divide between these 2 sectors is poor or nonexistent. Compounding the overall shortage of CAPs potentially available to collaborate with PCPs, those who are available are inadequately paid for the work done outside traditional office-based practice.

As discussed later in this article, a major feature of collaborative child and adolescent psychiatry practice is the practice of accepting new patient referrals from a PCP and referring some of these patients back to the PCP for continued management. This practice naturally results in an increase in the percentage of new patient visits relative to follow-up visits in the child psychiatry practice. Unfortunately, this threatens a reduction in practice revenue for the child psychiatrist because the increased amount of work associated with new patient evaluations is not adequately covered by insurance reimbursement. Behavioral health managed care entities typically require that psychiatrists use the CPT Psychiatry and Psychology Specialty Codes (series 908xx) rather than the CPT Evaluation/Management (E/M) Codes (series 992xx) used by any other medical specialist. Unlike E/M codes, the Psychiatry/Psychology Specialty Codes are not graded according to levels of complexity or time. As a result, child psychiatrists are unable to account for the increased time and effort associated with the frequently complex and multifaceted nature of their psychiatric evaluations. For example, an evaluation of a new patient in a regular outpatient office for a complex mental health problem would earn 6.28 RVUs[a] for a child psychiatrist using an E/M code (99245, high-level consultation, new or established patient). The same service would only earn 4.24 RVUs if the visit was coded with the allowable specialty code (90801).[8] Within these reimbursement conditions, there is an incentive for psychiatrists to see a high volume of established patients for brief follow-up visits with minimal time set aside for coordination with PCPs, rather than frequent new patient evaluations.

Most CPT codes apply to professional work provided for a patient who is physically present in the care setting (ie, face-to-face services) and insurers are accustomed to paying for these services. Collaboration between PCPs and psychiatrists often require communication activities performed *without the presence* of the patient or the patient's family, not necessarily associated with a patient visit. Non–face-to-face or indirect services, particularly those not associated with an office visit, are rarely paid by insurers, even if CPT codes are published and have assigned RVUs. For example, the Care Plan Oversight code (99339/99340) may apply to a telephone call from a psychiatrist to a PCP in certain limited circumstances; however, this code is not routinely covered under most insurance plans. Beyond the minimal "post-service" work included in the psychiatric specialty codes, telephone calls are not ordinarily eligible for reimbursement within most plans. Many plans similarly do not pay for team medical conferences among professionals involved with the child's care, communication with other medical and nonmedical professionals, including consultants, teachers, and therapists, nor many other indirect aspects of collaborative care for children (eg, care plan oversight, health risk assessment, and so forth).

There are additional barriers to collaborative models involving the colocation of behavioral health providers under the supervision of CAPs within pediatric primary care settings. According to the well-established practice of physicians employing allied medical professionals such as nurse practitioners and physician assistants to see patients in their offices under their supervision, there are so-called "incident to" standards under Medicare that allow physicians to bill for these services. Even though services that could be provided by advanced practice psychiatric nurses, psychologists, and social workers employed to work in PCP offices would meet these "incident to" standards, insurance plans generally do not allow this type of billing even though it is routinely allowed for analogous medical services.

---

[a] Reimbursement rates are generally set by insurance companies to be proportional to units called Relative Value Units (RVUs) within a system managed by the federal government entitled the Resource Based Relative Value Scale (RBRVS).

Increasing the opportunities for collaborative care between primary medical providers and child psychiatrists will necessitate advocacy by both groups to ensure more equitable payment for child psychiatry specialty services, increased reimbursement for non–face-to-face services for both psychiatrists and the primary care physicians, and improved support for colocated models involving allied behavioral health professionals.[9]

TRANSFORMING TRADITIONAL CHILD AND ADOLESCENT PSYCHIATRY PRACTICE TO INCORPORATE PRIMARY CARE COLLABORATION

Regardless of the size and complexity of the child psychiatry practice, change can be a very difficult process. If one accepts the premise that effective collaboration with pediatric primary care adds significant net value to psychiatric services for children and adolescents, then this process of change may naturally be considered a quality improvement initiative, and standard quality improvement methodology could be used to excellent advantage.

The Deming Cycle, otherwise known as the Plan-Do-Check-Act or PDCA cycle, has become a well-established methodology for quality and process improvement.[10] This methodology is a recurrent, iterative process: (1) Plan—define a problems or opportunities, identify a concrete achievable change in practice to address it; (2) Do—Implement the change, initially on a small scale; (3) Check—collect and analyze data to assess the impact of the change on the initial problem or opportunity; (4) Act—adopt the change, increase the scale of the change, discontinue it, or begin the cycle again with renewed planning.

During the initial planning, practices need to consider the purpose of collaboration with primary care and how that fits in with their own professional goals. Practices ultimately must decide what features of collaborative practice they would like to implement. For consideration in planning, a developmental model of 3 progressively intensive levels of collaboration with primary care is proposed here. Practices may begin with the initial level, focused on improving clinical communication with pediatricians. As they wish, they may progress to a deeper level of collaboration focusing on the enhancement of referral relationships and offering consultative services. Finally, a more systematic model of collaboration including reliable systems for delivery of various levels of consultation, care coordination, education, and guidance with screening and disease management is described. Tactics for implementation and methods for evaluating the impact of these tactics are suggested as examples for use within PDCA cycles.

LEVEL I: IMPROVING COMMUNICATION WITH PEDIATRIC PRIMARY CARE PROVIDERS

Effective communication is the cornerstone of all collaboration. Although there may certainly be some CAPs who maintain excellent levels of communication with their colleagues in primary care, many pediatricians report the experience of inadequate response to phone calls and a general lack of correspondence from CAPs.

Child psychiatrists are well aware of the importance of safeguarding the privacy and confidentiality of information associated with mental health treatment. Even though the Health Insurance Portability and Accountability Act of 1996 (HIPAA)[11] permits medical providers to share protected health information without specific authorization for the purpose of coordination of care and consultation, mental health providers often consider themselves obligated to require a special release of information to communicate with colleagues. In any case, the protection of confidentiality is rarely a valid reason for failure to communicate with PCPs. If the CAP feels that a release of information is necessary, then this should be routinely included in the initial packet of paperwork that new patients are asked to fill out at the first appointment.

Communication processes between physicians may be divided into 2 categories: (1) synchronous communication: this includes communication with parties present at the same time such as in-person conversation, telephone conversation, video conferencing, instant message, web paging; (2) asynchronous communication: this is a broad category that includes letter writing, email, and text messages, as well as transmitting or sharing medical records.

Telephone conversations are the most likely form of synchronous communication between PCPs and CAPs, although within integrated systems or large group practices, web paging technologies may be useful for the immediate communication of short messages. Although telephone communication is relatively inefficient and may be disruptive, it is often useful for rapidly exchanging ideas and joint problem solving. For example, a clinical issue discussed in a 5-minute phone conversation could otherwise require 4 or 5 lengthy email exchanges. Differences in office management and workflow between PCP and child and adolescent psychiatry practices represent obstacles to synchronous communication. In the primary care setting, physicians have patients in multiple examination rooms, and patients are accustomed to PCPs and their nursing staff coming in and out of the room during the office visit. Pediatricians usually instruct their staff to "pull" them from a room if a phone call comes in from another physician. In contrast, in the mental health setting, CAPs usually have a single office in which they see patients and families, one at a time. Patients expect and psychiatrists try to ensure for the patient to receive their undivided attention for the duration of the office visit. As a result, it would be disruptive for a CAP to be immediately available to take routine phone calls from PCPs. On the other hand, PCPs should be able to expect a voice message to result in a same-day return phone call and, in the case of an urgent issue regarding a shared patient, it is reasonable for a PCP to expect to reach a CAP immediately. Tactics to improve management of incoming telephone calls from PCPs include: (1) establishing a policy for same-day return of calls from PCPs and tracking compliance with the policy; (2) modifying outgoing voice-mail messages or answering service protocols to include an emergency contact procedure for use by PCPs.

Asynchronous communication such as sending messages or documentation electronically or by mail is the customary method of keeping PCPs informed of the current status of mental health issues and their treatment for patients. The common practice of relying on parents to serve as the messenger for conveying information between providers is unreliable, and may result in errors that can endanger patient safety. Information from CAPs about psychiatric medications, psychiatric diagnoses, treatment plans, and laboratory results is vitally pertinent to PCPs in performing well-child visits, monitoring chronic health conditions, preventing drug interactions, and evaluating new physical health symptoms. For the practice of transmitting information regarding mental health treatment to become routine, tactics must become systematic, be integrated into the workflow of the CAP, and require minimal additional effort beyond the CAP's ordinary documentation practices. Relevant office support staff accordingly must be involved in the planning of the communication. Routine office procedures for registration should include informing new patients of the practice of corresponding with PCPs and making sure that accurate PCP contact information is collected. Until child psychiatric treatment records become integrated into a shared electronic medical record system, the transmission of this information will require an additional step beyond the original documentation of the treatment.

The simplest method for keeping PCPs informed, often used by other medical specialists, is to automatically "cc" the initial evaluations and psychiatric progress notes to the PCP. If the CAP is providing weekly psychotherapy, this practice would be excessive; but, for periodic psychiatric follow-up, a copy of a concise progress note summarizing current status of symptoms, pertinent findings, and changes to the treatment plan could be a perfect vehicle for communication to the PCP. Of course notes must be legible and concise, avoiding excessive detail, speculation, or judgmental remarks.

A brief communication form is an alternative method for providing PCPs with information. The actual paper form or electronic template should be readily available on the desktop and should include fields for entering a problem list, psychiatric diagnosis, clinical status, a list of current treatments including medication information, and a field for additional information or questions. The form should be brief and easy to complete, to improve the likelihood of it being filled out by the CAP and being actually read by the PCP.

According to PDCA process improvement methodology, after implementation of initial tactics, the next step is to evaluate the implementation to assess whether the implementation was successful and to identify lessons learned. Improving telephone call response times is difficult to measure unless timed telephone logs for incoming messages and outgoing calls are maintained. Another approach for assessing implementation of a new policy regarding responding to PCP phone calls is to assess the satisfaction of the CAPs in the practice with the new guidelines. Questions could be asked regarding the frequency of PCP calls, the degree to which CAPs have been able to respond to them on the same day, the usefulness of the conversations with PCPs, and the frequency and appropriateness of the emergency calls from PCPs. The effectiveness of policies and procedures for routinely sending clinical information to PCPs could be easily assessed through periodic chart reviews as well as surveys of CAPs in the practice regarding the ease and convenience of using new communication forms. Of course, the most ambitious method of assessing tactics for improving communication would be a survey of PCPs to assess their satisfaction with the information received from the CAPs. This approach would most likely be feasible only for large systems with dedicated quality improvement staff.

LEVEL II: PROVIDING SERVICES THAT ARE RESPONSIVE TO THE NEEDS OF PRIMARY CARE PROVIDERS

Over time, as a traditional child psychiatry practice becomes fully established, relatively few new patient appointments are offered. Child psychiatric illnesses are often chronic, and one's practice becomes full with patients who are in maintenance phases of treatment or long-term psychotherapy. Such a practice is of little use to the pediatrician on the "front line" of the health care system. Practices striving to have a higher level of collaboration with pediatric PCPs may choose to develop strategies to more readily accept referrals from their colleagues in primary care.

As an initial step, a child and adolescent psychiatry practice would create a block of time in the weekly schedule and designate this time for new patient referrals from pediatricians. As noted, there is not much time available for new patients in a fully established practice, therefore it will be necessary to begin with a small block of time, perhaps accommodating 1 to 2 extra new patients per week. In a fully established practice, accepting additional patients would ordinarily increase the workload of the practice beyond the available time. Several tactics to prevent this may consequently be considered.

One tactic would be to define these extra new patient slots as consultation appointments. In accepting a referral for outpatient consultation, it is important for there to be an efficient triage process designed to identify the question for the consultation, and to ensure that both the referring PCP and the patient and family understand the time-limited nature of the service being offered. The triage process should also be aimed at selecting referrals for whom a consultation, rather than treatment directly by a child psychiatrist, is needed. Consultations are most useful for diagnostic clarification of patients whom the pediatrician will be able to treat in the primary care setting. Otherwise, the consultation may include (1) recommendations for further referral to specialists, (2) practical advice regarding how to access an often poorly coordinated array of community resources, and (3) suggestions regarding medical interventions that the PCP could provide on an interim basis. Even though the PCP may have ideally preferred to make a treatment referral to the CAP practice, in many cases, a 1- to 2-visit consultation including effective communication can be useful to the pediatrician and the patient.

Another tactic for preventing the practice from growing out of control in the context of increased new patient slots is to increase the turnover of the practice. This increase could be accomplished by implementing another feature of collaborative practice: a process for referring patients back to the PCP for maintenance treatment after the initial period of stabilization. Again, there needs to be understanding and approval of this process by the patient, family, and PCP at the outset of treatment. The complexity and severity of the patient's illness needs to be within the comfort level of the PCP. In addition, there must be an understanding that the patient will be accepted by the CAP for return consultation or treatment if questions arise or if the patient becomes unstable.

Implementing a plan to accept increased frequency of referrals, especially consultations, from PCPs, and to refer patients back to PCPs after stabilization, will call for a joint planning session with PCPs to negotiate mutual expectations and responsibilities. Starting small, with just one pediatric practice, is prudent. Growth can occur in successive PDCA cycles if the implementation is successful. Principles of effective communication with PCPs discussed in the previous section must be maintained diligently. Consultation letters must be timely and concise. Clinical documentation and a transfer note must accompany referrals of patients back to the pediatrician.

Continuing with the PDCA model of process improvement, to "check" the impact of these implementation tactics, indicators could include numbers of new patients seen during a specified time frame in comparison to a similar time frame prior to the implementation, patient and PCP satisfaction with the service, and child psychiatrist and staff satisfaction with the new process. It is also useful to include cost and revenue impact of the process as indicators. The child psychiatrist may find it interesting and worthwhile to see a higher volume of patients in more brief consultative and stabilization services, and enjoy the collegiality of the collaborative relationship with the pediatrician. The process alternatively may require various types of troubleshooting. For example, the relationship with the pediatrician may not be going smoothly, and mutual expectations may need to be renegotiated as a subsequent PDCA cycle is begun. Depending on reimbursement rates for consultation and increased time required for documentation and communication, there may be a positive or negative effect on hourly practice revenue. Keeping the initial implementation to a small scale minimizes the financial risk. In subsequent PDCA cycles, tactics to improve financial performance may be planned, such as streamlining documentation and communication, optimizing coding and billing processes, or renegotiating managed care contracts. Ensuring financial viability is a prerequisite for expansion and growth of these new services.

Additional Collaboration Tactics

Colocation

Some large pediatric primary care practices and multi-specialty group practices have chosen to engage CAPs or other children's mental health providers to work directly within or adjacent to primary care office suites. Having clearly identified specialty mental health providers working in such proximity sends a clear signal to children and families that the pediatrician considers mental health to be an ordinary part of primary care. The proximity also enables frequent informal curbside consultations, initial introductions of wary patients to mental health providers, and fluid transitions of care between specialist and PCP. Shared records may be used to further enhance communication. Although colocation is often not feasible because of space limitations and differing facility and practice support needs of child psychiatry practices, when possible, it can be extremely opportune for collaboration. It should be noted that it is possible for child psychiatrists to carry on a traditional or non-collaborative practice model, working in parallel with PCPs within a pediatric office suite. Collaborative processes do not automatically occur in a colocation environment; planning and implementation steps will continue to be required in order for the collaboration to flourish.

Telemedicine

For large sparsely populated areas, telemedicine technology is being used to make child and adolescent psychiatry services more accessible to children and families. In particular, CAPs use interactive video technology for clinical communication and examination of patients over long distances. In addition, this technology may be used to allow CAPs to remotely participate in case conferences and staff meetings. When necessary, telemedicine procedures have been found to be feasible for these functions and a useful tool for collaboration with pediatric PCPs over long distances. Similar to colocation, telemedicine procedures do not in themselves constitute collaborative practice. The technology brings patients and providers together over long distances; however, protocols for communication, implementing clinical recommendations, and follow-up need to be negotiated.

LEVEL III: SYSTEMIC COLLABORATION WITH PRIMARY CARE

With the development of productive collaborative relationships with selected primary care practices through improvement in communication practices, effective referral processes, and the regular offering of consultation services, CAP practices may wish to develop the capacity to replicate these relationships with PCPs throughout their region. CAPs may also wish to bring the capacity for consultation to a sufficient scale to reliably respond to the needs of a population in a geographic area. This type of expansion represents a transformation of a set of services into a program or system. Expanding collaborative services to such a scale is an ambitious initiative requiring extensive planning, dedicated resources, and a team-based approach. Also, special funding mechanisms are required to support the significant proportion of nonbillable services and infrastructure necessary for such a program.

A current example of this type of program, the Massachusetts Child Psychiatry Access Project (MCPAP), was funded directly from the Massachusetts state budget. Launched in June of 2005, MCPAP set up teams of children's mental health professionals in each of 6 regions blanketing the entire state.[12] The MCPAP teams were designed to respond to mental health needs of children in the primary care setting by providing primary care practices with rapid access to consultation, education, and care coordination services. Teams led by CAPs sought to enroll all pediatric primary care practices in their regions for participation. The vast majority of pediatric PCPs in the state have enrolled, covering 95% of the total population of children and adolescents. Each team operates a hotline, allowing PCPs to speak with a CAP or licensed child and family therapist within minutes. This initial telephone consultation not only provides practical advice and clinical education to the PCP at the point of care but also serves as the front end of a system offering direct clinical evaluation of children and adolescents, service finding/care coordination, mental health screening consultation, and brief interim psychotherapy for patients who are waiting for care. The teams consult on patients of enrolled pediatric PCPs of any age, regardless of insurance. Teams also provide child and adolescent psychiatry Continuing Medical Education programs for PCPs in their region. The program regularly communicates with enrolled PCPs regarding breaking developments in the field of children's mental health. The program has supported the implementation of state-wide mental health screening initiatives. In addition, the program has conducted pilot projects to provide consultation to public schools and to assist primary care practices in implementing a best-practice guideline for the evaluation and management of adolescent depression in primary care, the GLAD-PC.[13]

A regional system supporting the delivery of collaborative child psychiatry services for all children regardless of payer source is, by definition, a public health initiative and consequently requires government sponsorship, supported ideally by a blending of public and commercial insurance funding. To build support for such a system a coalition of CAPs, pediatricians, consumer advocates, and other stakeholders can raise public awareness regarding the importance of children's mental health. Addressing the urgency of the problem of inadequate access to care, and engaging health policy makers in discussions exploring potential solutions such as a collaborative care system can be a proactive advocacy strategy. Commercial health insurance plans, accountable to their members and purchasers for inadequate accessibility of mental health services, must be similarly engaged in these discussions and encouraged to support the development of the system. Although stymied by state fiscal challenges amid currently adverse economic conditions, advocates will find themselves in the company of a growing health care reform movement, emphasizing the importance of coordination of care and collaboration between PCPs and specialists as strategies for improving the quality and reducing unnecessary cost in health care.

SUMMARY

Regardless of pediatricians' lack of confidence in their training for primary management of mental health conditions, it must be acknowledged that they are already providing care for a large proportion of children with mental illness. In contrast, CAPs working in traditional practice models treat only a small fraction of children with significant psychiatric illness. Through the development of collaborative practices, CAPs enhance the ability of PCPs to respond effectively to children's mental health problems early in their course, thereby multiplying the impact of their unique skills. Collaborative practices with primary care allow CAPs to be involved in mental health prevention, to enjoy productive and collegial relationship with their pediatric colleagues, and to bridge historical and cultural divides between the mental health system and the general health care system. The presence of child psychiatrists in mainstream community systems such as primary care also serves to reduce the stigma associated with mental health problems. Incremental adoption of collaborative features in CAP practices through quality improvement methodology minimizes the risk associated with changes in clinical process, and can begin immediately for those CAPs who believe that this work is urgently needed in their community.

REFERENCES

1. Burns BJ, Costello EJ, Angold A, et al. Children's mental health service use across service sectors. Health Aff 1995;14(3):147–59.
2. Owens PL, Hoagwood K, Horwitz SM, et al. Barriers to children's mental health services. J Am Acad Child Adolesc Psychiatry 2002;41(6):731–8.
3. Horwitz SM, Kelleher KJ, Stein R, et al. Barriers to the identification and management of psychosocial issues in children and maternal depression. Pediatrics 2007;119(1):e208–18.
4. Leaf PJ, Owens PL, Leventhal JM, et al. Pediatricians' training and identification and management of psychosocial problems. Clin Pediatr 2004;43(4):355–65.
5. US Department of Health and Human Services, Center for Disease Control and Prevention. The role of the primary health care provider in children's developmental health. Available at: www.cdc.gov/ncbddd/child/screen_provider.htm. Accessed August 10, 2009.
6. Homer CJ, Klatka K, Romm D, et al. A review of the evidence for the medical home for children with special health care needs. Pediatrics 2008;123(2): e922–37.
7. Beebe M, Dalton JA, Espronceda M. Current procedural terminology 2009, professional edition. Chicago (IL): American Medical Association; October, 2008.
8. American Academy of Pediatrics, Practice Management Online. Improving mental health services in primary care: reducing administrative and financial barriers to access and collaboration: background article. Available at: practice. aap.org/content.aspx?aid=2775. Accessed August 10, 2009.
9. American Academy of Child and Adolescent Psychiatry, Committee on Health Care Access and Economics, American Academy of Pediatrics Task Force on Mental Health. Improving mental health services in primary care: reducing administrative and financial barriers to access and collaboration. Pediatrics 2009;123(4):1248–51.
10. Deming WE. Out of the crisis. Cambridge (MA): MIT Press; 1986.
11. US Dept of Health and Human Services. Summary of the HIPAA privacy rule. Available at: www.hhs.gov/ocr/privacy/hipaa/understanding/summary/index.html. Accessed August 10, 2009.
12. Massachusetts Child Psychiatry Access Project: connecting primary care with child psychiatry. Available at: www.mcpap.org. Accessed August 10, 2009.
13. Zuckerbrot RA, Cheung AH, Jensen PS, et al. Guidelines for adolescent depression in primary care (GLAD-PC). Pediatrics 2007;120(5):e1299–326.

Expanding the Vision: The Strengths-Based, Community-Oriented Child and Adolescent Psychiatrist Working in Schools

Avron Kriechman, MD*, Melina Salvador, MA, Steven Adelsheim, MD

KEYWORDS

- Children • Adolescents • Psychiatry • School mental health
- Community-oriented approach • Strength-based

For over a century, advocates of school mental health programs have recognized the intrinsic relationship between student mental health, child development, and school performance. School mental health programs have evolved within the context of various social movements, stressing equal educational opportunities for all youth in a supported, shared, and free learning environment. These efforts have the unique potential to address barriers to learning that so often prove devastating to young people in the United States, including "poverty, racism, gender discrimination, and disability."[1]

A BRIEF OVERVIEW OF RECENT DEVELOPMENTS IN SCHOOL MENTAL HEALTH SERVICES

By the middle of the twentieth century, the mental health needs of students were characteristically addressed on a case-by-case basis through the combined efforts of teachers, guidance counselors, school nurses, school psychologists, school social workers and, rarely, school psychiatrists. This service delivery model, essentially limited to assessment and intervention with individual students, has expanded to include other efforts, such as: (1) the linkage of the students and their families to Community Mental Health Centers, with the additional mandates of prevention and facilitating changes in the school culture; (2) the establishment of School-Based Health Centers (SBHCs) (wherein on-site primary care and mental health care

Department of Psychiatry, Center for Rural and Community Behavioral Health, University of New Mexico, MSC 09 5030, 1 University of New Mexico, Albuquerque, NM 87131-0001, USA
* Corresponding author.
E-mail address: akriechman@salud.unm.edu (A. Kriechman).

Child Adolesc Psychiatric Clin N Am 19 (2010) 149–162
doi:10.1016/j.chc.2009.08.005
1056-4993/09/$ – see front matter © 2010 Elsevier Inc. All rights reserved.
childpsych.theclinics.com

providers, working either for the school or a community agency, address both the health and mental health care needs of students); (3) Expanded School Mental Health Programs (providing a broad range of screening, prevention, assessment, and intervention services for regular and special education students); (4) Full Service Schools (coordinating and integrating a host of community services to offer students and their families a broader range of health care, mental health care, social and support services); and (5) Comprehensive School Approaches (system-wide efforts at school reform to provide mental health supports for all students). These new models of school mental health services provision create new opportunities for the child and adolescent psychiatrist working in the schools.

THE ROLE OF THE PSYCHIATRIST IN SCHOOL MENTAL HEALTH

Even though child psychiatry emerged decades ago, the role of the child and adolescent psychiatrist in the school mental health setting has yet to be clearly and formally articulated. The role any individual child and adolescent psychiatrist takes in the school mental health setting will depend on many factors including, but not limited to, what type of work is appealing to the individual, what training he or she has received, what type of work is available, the climate in the school mental health setting, and the support—systematic, administrative, or community based—that is provided. The task then becomes finding creative and systematic approaches that optimize community and individual strengths, while also meeting the needs of the particular school district and limiting the impact of bureaucratic, financial, and systems barriers.

The lack of clearly defined roles for child psychiatrists in the schools can and does present difficulties for integrating this specialty into this particular setting. At the same time, this lack of clarity offers an opportunity to set up context-specific, flexible collaborations to identify appropriate ways to integrate psychiatry into the school mental health setting that are culturally/setting appropriate, responsive to the needs of the community, and collaborative in nature. In the description of the Massachusetts, University of Maryland, and Center for Rural and Community Behavioral Health (CRCBH) models, the authors hope to communicate the considerable value child and adolescent psychiatrists can bring to school mental health settings, as well as some of the theoretical approaches that optimize this integration.

PSYCHIATRISTS AS CONSULTANTS IN THE SCHOOL

Perhaps the most typical way child and adolescent psychiatrists have been integrated into school mental health programs is as consultants. For decades the experts in mental health consultation in the schools, namely Berkovitz, Berlin, and Caplan, have advocated for psychiatrists to take an active and collaborative role in school mental health through ongoing interaction between 2 professional persons: the specialist consultant psychiatrist and the consultee (the school professional).[2] In this consultative model the professional responsibility remains with the consultee. Articulated most clearly in the Berlin model is the idea that the consultant can most effectively help children in schools by helping school professionals with their own internal difficulties, anxieties, and skills.[3] The Berkovitz model of professional-to-professional consultation in the schools highlighted the importance of cross-disciplinary communication skills in addition to specialty clinical knowledge when working in schools.[4] These models for mental health consultation have largely shaped the role of the child and adolescent psychiatrist in schools by: encouraging clinical as well as bureaucratic, administrative, and systems consultation with educators and other school professionals; fostering collaboration and communication across disciplines;

and demonstrating the importance of children's mental wellness for the success of the learning environment.

THE DOMINANT STORY OF THE SCHOOL-BASED PSYCHIATRIST

The path of least resistance for the child and adolescent psychiatrist involved in school mental health programs is providing what the American Academy of Pediatrics School Mental Health Policy Statement describes as the third tier of school mental health services: care for those with severe mental disorders.[5] In this instance, the child and adolescent psychiatrist functions primarily as diagnostician and psychopharmacologist. This psychiatrist may consult with providers who care for students on-site in schools or SBHCs, or provide these services directly in one of these school settings. Consultation to and supervision of primary care providers in schools (such as school nurses or nurse practitioners, physician assistants, or physicians working in a SBHC) is frequently limited to the indications for and management of psychotropic medications. Consultation with other behavioral health providers may often involve the coordination, rather than the integration, of psychopharmacological and psychotherapeutic interventions. At times, psychotropic medications are prescribed directly by the child and adolescent psychiatrist. The child and adolescent psychiatrist's input regarding the nature and course of psychotherapy, educational placement, and classroom management is often minimal, and generally considered outside the scope of the his or her responsibilities or expertise. The child and adolescent psychiatrist's connection to and collaboration with parents, families, and school-based providers is often limited to psychoeducation regarding the diagnosed disorders and their medication management, which may be the only form of mental health care provided. The psychiatrist's efforts are targeted to a select few of those most in need rather than the needs of the wider community of students, families, schools, and the additional school-based primary care and behavioral health providers who serve them.

The limited number and availability of child and adolescent psychiatrists,[6] the chronically unmet needs of students with serious mental illness, the relatively high cost of child psychiatrists to agencies and schools, and other systemic factors reinforce this dominant cultural narrative of the "appropriate" role for the child and adolescent psychiatrist: psychopharmacologist of the severely mentally ill or specialist consultant to generalist providers. Though appropriate in some ways, this limits the impact child and adolescent psychiatrists may have in the school mental health setting and may reduce job satisfaction, further compromising schools in their efforts to recruit and retain child and adolescent psychiatrists to work with students, families, educators, and school health professionals.

EVOLUTION BEYOND: CONTEMPORARY SCHOOL MENTAL HEALTH PROGRAMS

School mental health is undergoing a priority shift away from a model of child and adolescent psychiatrist as exclusively consultative or medication management for those most in need to an approach that can more adequately contribute to the provision of comprehensive and far-reaching mental health service in the schools. This shift is largely due to the recognition that there is a tremendous gap between the mental health needs of children and adolescents in the United States and the care they receive.[7] One study found that only 21% of children who need mental health evaluations receive services, and that this unmet need is particularly pronounced for Latinos and the uninsured.[8] It is widely acknowledged by the Surgeon General's Report on Mental Health, as well as other reports, that only a small percentage of young people with mental health problems receive the care they need, and most of these services are provided in a school setting.[9,10]

In fact, the development of SBHCs was predicated on this knowledge that health services need to be available in schools because "that is where kids are." In 2003 the President's New Freedom Commission specifically identified providing mental health services in schools as a critical part of building a successful mental health system for youth.[11]

Optimizing and facilitating the use of all available resources through the school is critical, especially at a time when mental health resources are scarce, there is a dearth of child and adolescent psychiatrists, and many children and their families have little or no access to care outside of the school setting. Important social movements in the fields of mental health and education call for a shift to less rigidly defined roles of "specialist," "expert," or "professional." This shift allows for the incorporation of parents, children, community members, and other social support persons into the consultation as experts where and when appropriate, and has the potential to best use existing resources in communities. Although a majority of schools throughout the United States still do not have the capacity to provide mental health services to their students in any manner, let alone in a comprehensive way, some programs are making innovative strides.

This shift to more comprehensive school-based mental health care bringing together multiplying partners including child and adolescent psychiatrists has been successfully articulated by various programs throughout the nation that are committed to this issue. The University of Maryland School Mental Health Program and the Massachusetts Child Psychiatry Access Project (MCPAP) are 2 examples. The University of Maryland School Mental Health Program brings together the Baltimore City Public School system and the Child and Adolescent Psychiatry training program at Maryland to address the dearth of psychiatric services available in the schools as well as the need for child and adolescent psychiatrists to be trained specifically how to work in the school setting (http://medschool.umaryland.edu/community/mental_health.asp). Child and adolescent psychiatry fellows are incorporated as consultants in these expanded school mental health programs during the second year of their fellowship. In addition to their primary responsibilities of conducting assessments and medication management, fellows are also able to participate in co-leading groups, presentations to teachers/faculty and classrooms, school-wide activities, school meetings, and Individualized Education Program meetings. Integral to the success of the Maryland training program is the emphasis placed on incorporating an understanding of the community context for the fellow. To achieve this goal, trainees learn about the city of Baltimore and its culture, including discussion of issues related to gangs, substance abuse, and violence, but also community history, religion, and geography. The trainees meet with school administrators, parents, and students, and do home visits. The trainees are introduced to local key programs and resources, and have extensive discussions about how working in the schools is different than standard psychiatric care. The development of the Maryland program highlights the value for both the school and the trainee of incorporating psychiatry trainees into the school mental health system, while demonstrating the importance of setting a tone for real collaboration across disciplines and with youth, families, and community members, as well as the importance of preparing the fellows to be able to provide culturally appropriate consultation.

The MCPAP has joined together child and adolescent psychiatrists in partnership with professionals from other disciplines in their implementation of a wide-ranging psychiatric consultation project. This project is an effort to extend child psychiatric services to Primary Care Providers throughout the Commonwealth area. The Commonwealth is currently initiating special outreach to "school nurses, child-care providers, school districts, Head Start programs, Early Intervention Program providers, and other providers and clinicians who come into contact with children under the age of 21" regarding access to this program[12] as well as providing formal linkages to SBHCs. In addition to consultation, the program offers behavioral health training and continuing education, and has a freely accessible and informative Web site that provides information on current issues about child mental health issues, as well as links to the substantial online resources at http://schoolpsychiatry.org through one of the regional MCPAP programs. Focusing on the link between the primary care provider and the consulting child and adolescent psychiatrist, this program has enhanced the potential impact of the consultant by broadening psychiatric consultation services offered to best meet the needs of the presenting child and family. Consultation services range from answering a question from a primary care provider to accepting a referral for an acute psychopharmacologic or diagnostic consultation.

THE UNIVERSITY OF NEW MEXICO-CRCBH MODEL: THE COMMUNITY-ORIENTED CHILD AND ADOLESCENT PSYCHIATRIST WORKING IN SCHOOLS
Expanding and Reaching the Frontier

The University of New Mexico (UNM) Child Psychiatry Division has a long history of providing child and adolescent psychiatry support to schools. Beginning with early school consultation efforts led by Irving Berlin, MD, with later expansion to include support for schools via SBHCs, this program has had a commitment to community mental health support through the school setting for decades. The traditional school-based training component has involved placing second-year fellows in urban SBHCs to serve as consultants to the school health professionals and SBHC staff, while also seeing students and families directly on-site. In an effort to ensure the school based component is not just one more typical medication clinic in a more distant location, trainees have been supported, like those in Maryland, to spend time in the classroom, give presentations at the school, and learn the intricacies of the school culture while on-site in the school setting.

Almost every county in New Mexico is designated a mental health professions shortage area, with almost half the counties designated as "frontier," less than 6 people per square mile. When this reality is combined with the recognition that at last count there were only 5 child psychiatrists practicing statewide outside of the Albuquerque/Santa Fe corridor, the need to develop innovative models to support rural child mental health care statewide becomes clear. Several factors have come together to allow for the development of an innovative approach to rural school mental health program support that reaches statewide while sustaining this training initiative. One component allowing for the broader role of child and adolescent psychiatrists in supporting schools throughout New Mexico has come with the state's expanded commitment to supporting child and adolescent health care by increasing the number of SBHCs throughout New Mexico. Furthermore, New Mexico has expanded its priority focus on telehealth support through the use of federal and state funds to increase the telehealth network to better support SBHCs and rural primary care sites, along with the development of a state Telehealth Commission.

These system changes have allowed New Mexico and the CRCBH to apply for and receive both federal and state funds to implement a unique model of child and adolescent psychiatry school support through the use of telehealth technology (http://hsc.unm.edu/som/psychiatry/CRCBH/). As a result, the UNM Health Sciences Center school-based experience for child psychiatry trainees has expanded, providing simultaneous experiences in school mental health, rural/frontier health care, and telehealth program development. The experience of those involved in this child and adolescent school-based telepsychiatry program at CRCBH further suggests that more expansive functions for child and adolescent psychiatrist, involving the first tier of preventive mental health programs and services, and the second tier of targeted mental health services for those with mental health needs, are not only possible but desirable.[5]

The Community-Oriented Multidisciplinary Approach

The guiding theoretical model of the UNM-CRCBH program is a community-oriented approach whereby the consulting child and adolescent psychiatrist is included as a key member of a nonhierarchical multidisciplinary team. This team often includes family members and other essential social supports, and values the expertise each co-participant brings to the interaction. The model offers unique cross-training opportunities for all participants and supports open communication, empowerment, and sharing of knowledge. The model requires flexibility and its impact is enhanced by administrative, financial, and community-based support. Furthermore, this model offers a wide range of services to children and families, on-site primary care, and behavioral health providers and school professionals. In some instances, direct on-site services are provided to community mental health centers serving these students in the community. Given the critical mental health needs of students in rural and frontier areas of New Mexico, a major focus of the UNM-CRCBH program involves a community-oriented, strengths-based approach, through which greater possibilities for the role of the child and adolescent psychiatrist in the school mental health system have emerged.

The child and adolescent psychiatrists participating in the UNM-CRCBH School Telepsychiatry Program may be involved in one or more of the following: (1) direct service (primary responsibility for the prescription and management of psychotropic medication) to students diagnosed with severe mental disorders by means of telepsychiatry interviews of students with or without their families or providers; (2) case-based consultation, training, and supervision of school-based primary care providers regarding psychotropic medication; (3) case-based consultation, training, and supervision of school-based primary care and behavioral health care providers regarding the integration of psychotherapeutic and psychopharmacological interventions; (4) interdisciplinary case conferences involving educators, behavioral health care providers, or primary care providers with the aim of creating collaborative treatment plans and case management; (5) training sessions for educators, behavioral health care providers, or primary providers regarding screening, assessing, diagnosing, and treating mental disorders; (6) case-based telepsychiatry larger system interviews engaging students, families, peer supports, educators, and both school-based and community behavioral health or primary care providers in a conversation regarding a mutual agreed on course of action; (7) case-based larger system telepsychiatry interviews addressing and surmounting interdisciplinary, interagency, and community barriers to collaboration; and (8) case-based service delivery telepsychiatry consultations with the aim of creating a multifaceted, multisite, community-based system of care for students with mental health needs. The child and adolescent school telepsychiatry program may use illustrative case examples as a trigger for addressing and contributing to the revision of risk assessment, safety, suicide prevention, crisis intervention, critical incident, and confidentiality protocols within schools and school districts.

Effective Schools

Key to the breadth and depth of the child and adolescent psychiatrist's involvement is a guiding personal philosophy (based on supportive training) that embraces a nonhierarchical, trusting partnership with students, families, educators, primary care providers, and other behavioral health care providers, and an ability to assess, work with, and consult to larger systems of care.[13] Families and educators are seen as having unique insights, perspectives, competencies, and resources, being collaborators and cocreators of interventions and treatments. This view extends far beyond the bounds of families and educators as mere sources of history and information; it assumes "unique ways of cooperating" rather than resistance and noncompliance,[14] an outlook shared by national recovery and resiliency based models of consumer and family mental health care.[15] Behavioral health and primary care providers are seen as partners rather than competitors, valued for their expertise and experience rather than their discipline and degree. The community-oriented child and adolescent school psychiatrist engages in "therapeutic conversations" in which the language and understandings of student and family take precedence over the "expert" language and understandings of the "professionals."[16] The child and adolescent psychiatrist demonstrates respect, curiosity, and support for the particular strengths and stories of student and family, educators, and providers,[17] and is able to use[18] their narratives, beliefs, and experiences in the mutually collaborative creation of a plan of action embracing all of the settings in which the student lives. Within this framework, the child and adolescent psychiatrist is in the uniquely privileged position of integrating the physical with the psychological, the psychopharmacological with the psychotherapeutic, and the educational with the provision of physical and behavioral health care. The child and adolescent psychiatrist can "encourage consistent strategies that promote practice and reinforcement of social, emotional, and behavioral learning across contexts."[19] This focus can best be upheld within strengths-based therapeutic discussions which support and amplify educator-based conversations about activity, learning, and relationship strengths,[20] cocreating a developmentally grounded plan of action connecting home, school, and community. Maintaining a focus on the impact of mental health issues on the student's learning, academic performance, school behavior, and school attendance provides common ground for a discourse that best engages students, families, educators, and health care providers.

The guiding philosophy of this strengths-based, community-oriented, systemic telepsychiatry model corresponds well with the Effective Schools movement in education. Both advocate a shift from "deficit-based," "disease-based," and "fault-finding" methodologies to an approach that embraces the establishment of "collective trust" and "self and collective efficacy," and uses the findings of "positive psychology" and "positive organizational scholarship" to "engage" "multi-shareholders" in the articulation of "core purpose and values around teaching and learning."[21]

Building a Community of Care: A Strengths-Based Model

The community-oriented, strengths-based approach of both "effective schools" and the UNM-CRCBH school telepsychiatry program take a broader view of family and support systems, valuing and encouraging the active participation of families-of-choice (families that are constructed socially and culturally rather than biologically), peers, lay professionals, community volunteers, and others, opening the system to a chorus of voices. The following examples demonstrate the value added from this perspective. In each of the examples, the child and adolescent psychiatrists invited individuals who were identified by the student or family as essential supports to participate in the telehealth meeting event.

At one team meeting attended by a young woman's estranged parents, siblings, counselor, teacher, and boyfriend (identified by her as critical to her well-being), her boyfriend revealed that he had witnessed the murder of a close friend, stating that this experience provided him greater empathy and understanding regarding his girlfriend's exposure to the savage attack on her father that had traumatized everyone in the family.

In another telehealth meeting, a teacher's aide was invited to join the mother, teacher, social worker, and school psychologist. The aide was initially discounted by the school psychologist. However, after being acknowledged as "the expert" on the student's behavior by the student's mother and the psychiatrist, the aide revealed heretofore hidden and critical information regarding the nature of the student's difficulties.

One student had chosen the school bus driver to entrust her long history of victimization at the school—victimization intimately connected to her previously inexplicable attempts at self-injury. The bus driver shared with the providers how she had encouraged the student to attend the team meeting and secure the treatment she needed. Her story of how the bus driver engaged, joined, listened to, and supported this young woman created the foundation for the team's recommendations and plans.

In each of the examples here, having multiple voices not only offers new information and new understanding, but builds a more diverse and meaningful "community of concern" for students and the family, peers, educators, providers, and lay professionals attempting to support and assist them.[17]

Another benefit of this more all-embracing role for the child and adolescent psychiatrist is the potential for greater opportunities for engaging students, families, and educators who might otherwise decline an invitation to meet with someone seen as constructing a deficit-based assessment resulting in psychotropic medication as the main, if not sole, form of recommended treatment. Introduced to a community-oriented child and adolescent psychiatrist rather than a psychopharmacologist, students, families, and educators predisposed to reject psychotropic medications and pathologic descriptions may be more open to view medication as one of many potentially useful interventions. This framework also creates the space for a shared,[22] decisional balance-based[23] discussion in which the psychiatrist reviews potential pros and cons regarding medication and the beliefs and values related to them.

A crucial component of these strengths-based "therapeutic conversations"[16] involves the ongoing encouragement of feedback about what is useful and what works. Most psychiatrists in training are used to a top-down hierarchical model in which the psychiatrist prescribes and advises while everyone else listens. It is another matter altogether to be a coparticipant in a collaborative conversation, a source of information and expertise rather than an authority and team leader. It is therefore incumbent on the child and adolescent psychiatrist to invest in becoming well-versed in and respectful of the resources, diverse cultures, and local knowledge of the community in which student, family, and school are situated.

All of these efforts connect to a self-determined mandate regarding serving populations and communities rather than solely treating a select group of individuals requiring intensive intervention. It is helpful for the child and adolescent psychiatrist to have training in family, group, systems, and time-effective psychotherapies as well as policies, procedures, and programs regarding educational assessment and placement. UNM Child Psychiatry fellows participate in seminars in family and time-effective psychotherapy as well as telepsychiatry as an introduction to the skill set that is required. Strengths-based, community-oriented descriptions and ideally are not limited to one clinical rotation, but are part and parcel of the entire child and adolescent psychiatry training program, endorsed and used by teachers, supervisors, and colleagues throughout the course of the 2-year program and school-based programs as an introduction to the skill set that is required.

Modeling Flexibility and Transparency

It is important to model innovation and flexibility in training sessions, conferences, team meetings, and conversations so that a community of care is envisioned and co-determined as circumstances demand. For instance, the UNM child and adolescent school telepsychiatry program has involved peer educators, community gate-keepers,[24] security guards, bus drivers, cafeteria workers, teachers' aides, parent volunteers, consumer and community advocates, school administrators, and others when their pivotal role in screening, assessing, supporting, or advising students with mental health needs has emerged during the course of case-based conversations.

Flexibility is also modeled in the child and adolescent psychiatrist's response to the failure of videoconferencing technology or the difficulty of gathering everyone together at one site by arranging that participants connect (from work, school, home, or agency) by telephone conference call to those for whom videoconferencing is available. Working parents, for example, can more readily be involved in team meetings when they can join by conference call from their workplace rather than take time off work to join school-based providers in the school. This participation demonstrates the value placed on hearing everyone's voice, coincidentally deemphasizing the primacy placed on the limited availability and schedule (and higher cost) of the child and adolescent psychiatrist.

Another means of growing the audience of support for students, families, and schools involves making DVDs (or weblinks) to archived televideo training sessions, and encouraging those attending the live session to serve as discussants and facilitators for on-site follow-up sessions. This method expands the network of community advocates, peer counselors, community gatekeepers, and stakeholders in the promotion of mental health and wellness, and the prevention, screening, assessment, early intervention, and treatment of students with mental health needs. It is critical that such training sessions and workshops review general rather than case-based information, because even consciously deidentified case material is often identified in smaller communities.

Guidelines related to the procedures for obtaining consent for the telepsychiatry interview also support this overall philosophy of open communication, empowerment, and shared knowledge. Consent is to be obtained from the student and family in advance of the telepsychiatry interview. This consent occurs in the form of a conversation that stipulates treatment will not be withheld if the student and family decline the option of the televideo (or telephone) interview. The student and family are further informed that they may end the interview (either the video component or the interview altogether) at any point in time. The participants in the telepsychiatry interview are selected by the student and family (in some cases, the student may elect not to include the family in the initial interview).

This spirit of transparency is furthered by the psychiatrist's documentation of the telepsychiatry interview. The report is written with the intent that all present (student, family, supports, providers) are invited to read and discuss it, in the hope that it will further the collaborative conversation sparked by the telepsychiatry meeting. The report is seen as a vehicle to continue the conversation and open it up, rather than end the conversation through privileged information closed to all but a select few. Writing reports in this fashion also serves as a corrective against "expert," technical, or derogatory descriptions and characterizations. Students and parents codetermine what they wish to have the psychiatrist document, and what is to be shared with educational and health care providers. Without exception, families have asked for the full documentation of all diagnostic labels, assessments, and treatment recommendations. This transparency not only builds collective trust, but continues to reinforce the need for strengths-based, positive descriptions by all concerned for the student's welfare. The suggestion that the report may be shared by all present is given toward the close of each telepsychiatry meeting.

Expanding the Role of the Child and Adolescent Psychiatrist

The role of the child and adolescent psychiatrist in highlighting and cocreating community resources for intervention and treatment cannot be underestimated. School-wide programs that focus primarily on screening and assessment of students with mental health needs without the expansion of treatment capacity risk increasing demand with no supply.[25] This situation is demoralizing and disempowering for those advocating for students with mental health needs. Careful consideration must be given in matching screening to treatment, and the child and adolescent psychiatrist can play a critical role in reconfiguring existing community resources to better accommodate the increasing demand for mental health services. Examples of services to be encouraged include time-effective therapies, medication management groups, multiple family groups, psychoeducation groups, community-based peer support groups, and after-school activities that nurture social supports.

This enhanced role for the child and adolescent psychiatrist expands on the typical administrative functions inherent in the field. This multifaceted role for the child and adolescent psychiatrist working with schools on-site or via telepsychiatry also provides trainees a unique experience integrating many aspects of prevention, early assessment, early intervention, treatment, consultation-liaison, and interdisciplinary teamwork in one clinical rotation rather than one that is a psychopharmacology clinic, with the slight variation that it occurs through videoconferencing.

The UNM-CRCBH child and adolescent psychiatry program supports many of the objectives advanced by the American Academy of Child and Adolescent Psychiatry's Systems-Based Practice Educational Systems Objectives,[26] including developing the ability "to understand the socio-cultural milieu of the school" and develop "an empathetic understanding of the needs of youth, families, and educational providers." The child and adolescent psychiatry fellowship, however, cannot be the beginning of training in and socialization to this model. Trainees at all levels would ideally have ongoing cultural experiences in the community with students, parents, and teachers as their instructors. The trainees would be encouraged to honor the tradition and history of those individuals and communities with whom they connect. Their curiosity would be sparked by strengths, competencies, and expertise (rather than "expertise"). And they would learn how to listen, reflect, converse, and understand, rather than prescribe and ordain.

ADMINISTRATIVE ISSUES

The managerial alliance and psychological contract[27] between the community-oriented child and adolescent psychiatrist and the patients, families, schools, and agencies is exemplified in the interdisciplinary, collaborative, therapeutic conversation described earlier. For such a project, establishing the protocols for consultants and consultees regarding (1) roles, (2) responsibilities, (3) transparency of documentation and communication, (4) respect for the expertise and cultural diversity of all concerned, and (5) an emphasis on obtaining the consent and maintaining the confidentiality of the patients and their families clearly delineated the values, mandates, and vision of the project as well as the mutual obligations between the psychiatrist and providers in schools and health care agencies regarding the behaviors most productive of the goals of the project.

These protocols and procedures were established via lengthy discussions within the CRCBH telehealth team and by means of actual or virtual (video- or phone-conferencing) site visits with the target schools and agencies. The protocols and procedures also involve an active feedback loop between psychiatrist, consultees, patients, families, and the CRCBH telehealth team, including Customer and Provider Satisfaction Surveys. This emphasis on the management of change and the change process is mirrored in the flexible, adaptive menu of possible psychiatrist activities as interviewer and diagnostician, family/systems consultant, educator and trainer, and coparticipant in therapeutic conversations. This flexible, innovative, responsive approach is exemplified in using multiple modalities (telephone, televideo, and on-site) to widen the sphere of participants for any given conversational event, in the use of follow-up emails with evidence-based references of interest, and in the use of pre- and post-event phone calls. The pre-event phone call establishes the participants and basic structure for the upcoming meeting, providing the psychiatrist an opportunity to involve a broader community of support. The post-event phone call focuses on learning what worked and what did not, so as to continuously improve the nature and utility of the psychiatrist-system interaction. This process of open and ongoing communication between the psychiatrist and all concerned not only furthers therapeutic goals, but provides the information needed to monitor and adapt the structure and processes of the collaborative effort. Of note, the on-camera inclusion and active participation of psychiatric trainees demonstrates the UNM Department of Psychiatry's administrative support for the values and mission of the CRCBH project and the need for future psychiatrists to adopt those values in their own practice.

To provide the flexible, supportive model that allows for a collaborative partnership, a clear agreement surrounding the clinical and administrative responsibilities must be established. The CRCBH model of telehealth support for school programs comes from multiple federal, state, and local funding sources, but each clinical partnership has a contractual delineation of relationship and responsibilities. Within this contractual framework it is critical to clarify several components. One important aspect of this relationship, particularly when individual patients and connected family, friends, or school personnel are seen, requires clarification of who has ultimate responsibility for the clinical care of the patient. In the CRCBH model, the clinical contract clarifies the "consultant" role of the child psychiatrist, allowing for the ultimate clinical decision making to rest with the local provider, patient, and family. Consultation notes are delivered to the site through a variety of means, the site where the patient resides making sure that the notes reach the correct chart. Furthermore, for the patient's protection, the CRCBH program requires the informed consent of the patient and family before presentation of their "case" in all situations, even if not a face-to-face clinical visit. An understanding of the state law regarding both informed consent and confidentiality rights for minors is critical to ensuring the appropriate policies and consents are in place before developing these consent procedures. In addition, delineation of the availability of the child psychiatrist for urgent or emergent issues during the regular work week, as well as evenings and weekends, must be clarified contractually. Liability issues and malpractice coverage related to patient consultation and clinical responsibility must be clearly described in any contract, to ensure all involved are aware of and comfortable with their legal responsibilities.

THE POSSIBILITIES OF CHANGE

An expanded vision and role for the child and adolescent psychiatrist regarding school mental health requires administrative and financial support. This support is facilitated once it is realized that the limited time of the child and adolescent psychiatrist may easily be filled by direct service for a small number with severe mental illness and, therefore, may be best employed for maximum impact in the larger systems/community partnerships outlined earlier. One larger-systems interview may not only recruit a community of support and treatment for an individual student, but initiate a series of changes in the ways in which providers, educators, and families screen for, assess, and treat students with mental health needs. It is the experience of the UNM-CRCBH child and adolescent telepsychiatry program that a mission promoting the health of the school community is quickly welcomed and supported by students, families, schools, behavioral health providers, and primary care providers alike.

This programmatic emphasis on resiliency, recovery, self-efficacy, and agency is supported by recent Federal mandates laid out by the President's New Freedom Commission on Mental Health and others. Programs like the ones described in this article offer examples for how to operationalize the goals set forth by the Commission. Such programs have the potential to improve the quality of mental health care for children and adolescents precisely because they are transdisciplinary, located in schools, and strengths based; they integrate family, friends, and community, and emphasize sustainability and expansion through broad-based training.

Specific programmatic implementation details will depend on each community. For example, New Mexico uses telehealth because of the rural/frontier nature of the state and the need for broader outreach, given the lack of child and adolescent psychiatry statewide. In one survey primary care providers throughout New Mexico designated child psychiatry as their greatest need of all specialties. However, the model described here could be used effectively in urban settings as well with direct on-site participation of the child and adolescent psychiatrist with student, family, school, and community partners. The ability to allow parents and other attendees to participate by phone or other methods to help overcome barriers due to work or other obligations might still be considered in the urban implementation of such a model. In some urban communities, telehealth is even used within the same city for child and adolescent psychiatric support in local schools. Telehealth, in this instance, reduces local travel time for the heavily scheduled child and adolescent psychiatrist.[28]

The philosophical shift inherent in all the models described here for the child and adolescent psychiatrist must be reinforced in training programs. The skill development needed to work in school settings early and throughout training must be emphasized. One must continue to ensure that trainees understand the importance of the strengths-based recovery framework now part of the national and state mental health systems. The training experiences within the community for trainees to learn systematic approaches to mental health support must be provided for. Given the ongoing scare numbers, it is essential that residents be taught to be partners with their patients, families, school personnel, and primary care colleagues, thence to better meet the need for mental health support not only for individuals and families, but communities as a whole. If one has the therapeutic belief that "change is inevitable,"[14] not rare or merely possible, it follows that the role of the child and adolescent psychiatrist working with schools must support the shift "from problem to possibility,"[21] so both schools and the child and adolescent psychiatrists working with them are more "effective" in supporting students, families, and communities.

REFERENCES

1. Flaherty T, Osher D. History of school-based mental health services in the United States. In: Weist Mark D, Evans Steven, Nancy Lever, editors. Handbook of school mental health: advancing practice and research. New York: Kluwer Academic/Plenum Publishers; 2003. p. 11–22.
2. Caplan G. Types of mental health consultation. Am J Orthop 1963;33:470–81.
3. Berlin I. Mental health consultation to child-serving agencies as therapeutic intervention. In: Noshpitz JD, Harrison S, Call Justin D, editors. Basic handbook of child psychiatry: therapeutic interventions. New York: Basic Books; 1979. p. 353–64.
4. Berkovitz I. School interventions: case management and school mental health consultation. In: Sholevar GP, Benson RM, Blinder BJ, editors. Treatment of emotional disorders in children and adolescents. New York: Spectrum Publications; 1980. p. 501–20.
5. Committee on School Health. School-based mental health services. Pediatrics 2004;113:1839–45.
6. Thomas C, Holzer C. The continuing shortage of child and adolescent psychiatrists. J Am Acad Child Adolesc Psychiatry 2006;45(9):1–9.
7. Stephan SH, Weist M, Kataoka S, et al. Transformation of children's mental health services. Psychiatr Serv 2007;58(10):1330–8.
8. Kataoka S, Zhang L, Wells K. Unmet need for, the national institute of mental health care among U.S. children: variation by ethnicity and insurance status. Am J Psychiatry 2002;159:1548–55.
9. Rones M, Hoagwood K. School-based mental health services: a research review. Clin Child Fam Psychol Rev 2000;3(4):223–41.
10. Available at: http://www.surgeongeneral.gov/library/mentalhealth/home.html. Accessed April 03, 2009.
11. U.S. Department of Health and Human Services, Final report for the president's new freedom commission on mental health. Achieving the promise: Transforming mental health care in America. Pub no SMA-03-3831. Rockville (MD) 2003. Available at: http://www.mentalhealthcommission.gov/reports/reports.htm. Accessed April 03, 2009.
12. Available at: http://www.mass.gov/Eeohhs2/docs/masshealth/provlibrary/epsdt-cbh-fs2.pdf. Accessed April 03, 2009.
13. Imber-Black E. Families and larger systems: a family therapist's guide through the labyrinth. New York: The Guilford Press; 1988.
14. De Shazer S. Patterns of brief family therapy: an ecosystemic approach. New York: The Guilford Press; 1982.
15. U.S. Department of Health and Human Services. National consensus statement on mental health recovery. Washington DC. Available at: http://mentalhealth.samhsa.gov/publications/allpubs/sma05-4129/. Accessed April 03, 2009.
16. Anderson H, Goolishian H. Human systems as linguistic systems: preliminary and evolving ideas about the implications for clinical theory. Fam Process 1988;27:371–93.
17. White M, Epston D. Narrative means to therapeutic ends. New York: W.W. Norton & Company; 1990.

18. O'Hanlon, Hudson William. Taproots: underlying principles of Milton Erickson's therapy and hypnosis. New York: W.W. Norton & Company; 1987.

19. Paternite CE, Johnston TC. Rationale and strategies for central involvement of educators in effective school-based mental health programs. J Youth Adolesc 2005;34(1):41–9.

20. Fox J. Your child's strengths: discover them develop them use them. New York: Viking; 2008.

21. Daly AJ, Chrispeels J. From problem to possibility: leadership for implementing and deepening the processes of effective schools. J Effective Schools 2005; 4(1):7–25.

22. Deegan PE, Rapp C, Hotter M, et al. Best practices: a program to support shared decision making in an outpatient psychiatric medication clinic. Psychiatr Serv 2008;59(6):603–5.

23. Janis IL, Mann L. Decision making: a psychological analysis of conflict, choice, and commitment. New York: The Free Press; 1977.

24. Wyman PA, Brown CH, Inman J, et al. Randomized trial of a gatekeeper program for suicide prevention: 1-year impact on secondary school staff. J Consult Clin Psychol 2008;76(1):104–15.

25. US Preventive Task Force. Screening and treatment for major depressive disorder in children and adolescents: US Preventive Services Task Force recommendation statement. Pediatrics 2009;123(4):1223–8.

26. American Academy of Child and Adolescent Psychiatry. Systems-based practice: educational system. 2009. Working document to be available at: http://www.aacap.org/. Accessed April 03, 2009.

27. Cozza SJ, Hales RE. Leadership. In: Talbot JA, Hales RE, Keill SL, editors. Textbook of administrative psychiatry. 1st edition. Washington, DC: American Psychiatric Press; 1992. p. 31–58.

28. Bryant B. Telepsychiatry gets good reception with Texas high school students. Psychiatr News 2007;42(5):22.

Community Systems of Care for Children's Mental Health

Mark Chenven, MD[a,b,c],*

KEYWORDS

- Children's mental health • Systems of care • Wraparound
- Community psychiatry • Family-driven care

Although still a work in progress, the community systems of care model now serves as the conceptual framework defining the organization of public children's mental health and other social welfare programs for youth across the nation. The model now widely informs practice and planning efforts, even in locales lacking the resources or initiative to implement comprehensive program reform. Some communities have experienced an extensive revitalization of local public mental services because of system of care practice implementation. Core components of the model are its reliance on the constructs of the wraparound approach for supporting youth and families to succeed in community care, and its use of integrative interagency practices among relevant child-serving systems.[1]

The current state of system of care programming is a product of nearly 30 years of development within the public mental health arena, guided in large part by policy initiatives elaborated by the federal government. This policy effort has been shaped by a mixture of forces, including families, family advocates, mental health professionals, the social research community, and others. These constituencies have advocated for reorganized systems offering improved and expanded services, lobbied successfully for enabling legislation and funding, effected change through class action litigation at state and local levels, and conducted research and inquiry into system efficacy.

The system of care model of utilizing integrated interagency processes and wraparound services now represents the "community standard of care" for public mental health services. For child/adolescent psychiatrists (CAPs), this represents both an opportunity and a challenge. The clinical capabilities and multiple specialized skills of CAPs are sorely needed in these service systems, yet these clinicians (and other

[a] Division of Child and Adolescent Psychiatry, Department of Psychiatry, UCSD Medical School, 3030 Children's Way, Suite 111, San Diego, CA 92123, USA
[b] Vista Hill Foundation, 8787 Complex Drive, Suite 200, San Diego, CA 92123, USA
[c] Work Group on Community Systems of Care, American Academy of Child & Adolescent Psychiatry, 3615 Wisconsin Avenue, NE, Washington, DC 20016, USA
* Vista Hill Foundation, 8787 Complex Drive, Suite 200, San Diego, CA 92123.
E-mail address: mchenven@vistahill.org

Child Adolesc Psychiatric Clin N Am 19 (2010) 163–174
doi:10.1016/j.chc.2009.08.006
1056-4993/09/$ – see front matter © 2010 Published by Elsevier Inc.

childpsych.theclinics.com

professionals) must adjust their thinking and adapt their skill sets to work effectively within the paradigm and become familiar with its new approaches, environments, and service modalities.[2]

Public mental health systems operate in all states and in tribal and territorial jurisdictions pursuant to federal guidelines and funding mechanisms. Although the accessibility, focus, quality and efficacy of services provided vary considerably across local jurisdictions, these systems represent a core element of each community's and the nation's public health infrastructure. Financial support for these systems comes through federal grants, federal–state Medicaid partnership, state and local funding, user fees and, increasingly, from other child-serving agency sources.

THE SYSTEM OF CARE MODEL

Public mental health programs are responsible for providing care to children who have severely impairing acute and chronic mental health disorders. These programs give priority to those who do not have ready and adequate access to care because of socioeconomic challenge, and also to those involved with other child-serving public sector systems, such as child welfare, juvenile justice, special education, developmental disabilities, and substance abuse.

Working with these populations is challenging and complex, because mental health concerns often interface with a multiplicity of coexisting social, cultural and legal considerations. With its wraparound inspired methods, the system of care model represents an emerging yet well-defined approach to intervening in these complex situations on behalf of children who have significant mental health needs and on behalf of their families. The goals, most simply put, entail organizing services to address the needs and capacities of children and their families within a local community context in collaboration with other youth and family serving systems.

Although similar goals and strategies are applied in the private practice arena, in public sector activity, organizing services to achieve these goals incorporates new approaches in working with families and child-serving agencies. When implemented with fidelity to its core principles, systems of care have shown significantly positive outcomes in clinical, fiscal, and other domains,[3] and these modalities and approaches are becoming increasingly relevant to private practice settings and systems.

The Wraparound Approach to Services

Using an approach to fostering family and youth empowerment and capacity, known as the *wraparound process*, the system of care model has disseminated a broad array of new forms of intervention, including the activities of parent partnering, team decision making, strength-based care planning, paraprofessional mentoring, in-home respite, access to needed cash assistance, and other services and supports that may enhance the functioning of youth and families with complex needs. These new modalities supplement traditional professional continuum of care approaches, with outreach offered beyond clinic walls, at homes, and in community settings.[4]

The model encourages family-driven/youth-guided care, in which youth and their families more actively define their objectives, direct care decision making, and participate assertively in treatment and service deliberations. Special attention is paid to relevant community and cultural resources and supports. At a macro level, the model also requires family and youth participation in guiding policy and system evolution in local, state, and federal system deliberations.[5]

A hallmark of wraparound programming is the use of paraprofessional mentoring and support services that are delivered under clinically guided care management protocols and monitoring. Child and adolescent psychiatrists may play roles in wrap-around services through collaborative participation in direct service activities and participation in care management activities.

Integrative Interagency Practice

Given the multisystemic challenges and needs of youth served in public systems, the system of care model also fosters the integration of mental health services with other child-serving systems. The provision of mental health within school systems is perhaps the most obvious and widespread of these activities, with growing numbers of communities supporting school-based outpatient and day treatment services, in situ, allowing for better coordination among mental health workers and school staff. These programs help increase parental involvement with both educational services and mental health treatment.

Likewise, mental health programs for youth under the jurisdiction of Juvenile Court probation and child welfare systems are increasingly available. With awareness that foster children and delinquent youth have significantly higher rates of mental, psycho-social, and developmental vulnerability, many communities are increasingly investing resources to obtain mental health assessment and treatment for high-risk target populations as adjunctive elements in their core traditional service activities.[6]

Other interagency target populations, such as youth who have substance abuse problems and developmental disabilities, also receive collaborative mental health services because they have a higher prevalence of co-occurring mental health problems, although stigma, lack of capacity, and poor coordination continue to hamper optimal program and service development in these arenas.

With considerable promise, attention is increasing within the system of care movement on transition-age youth (TAY), youth aging out of the children's mental health system, and for preschool populations, with interest in developing service systems for younger children and their families within early childhood mental health (ECMH) systems of care.

Interagency integrative practice, as a core element of the system of care model, is actively promoting the long discussed but rarely achieved goal of providing genuine prevention and early intervention services.[7]

Outcomes Evaluation

Outcomes evaluations of system of care programs funded through the Substance Abuse, Mental Health Services Administration's (SAMHSA) Center for Mental Health Services' (CMHS) demonstration projects[8] describe findings of increased patient functionality, greater educational attainment, increased residential stability and reduced out-of-home placements, decreased caregiver stress, improved caregiver employment, and higher client satisfaction. Notable system outcomes have included an increased role of case management, the growing use of paraprofessional mentorship services, reductions in the use of residential and inpatient care, increased cultural competency amongst staff and evidence of earlier access to care.[9]

An increase of integrative practice and collaboration between distinct child-serving agencies is evident, including more collocation of mental health staff in other child-serving institutions and increased use of blended funding initiatives for collaborative programming efforts. The concept of "system-ness" has been proposed as an outcomes ideal for community mental health systems, which is a true system that provides accessible, effective, coordinated, culturally competent consumer-centric services and supports policy that optimizes the integrity and well-being of its children and families.

THE HISTORICAL CONTEXT

To appreciate the import of the system of care paradigm, it is helpful to briefly trace the evolution of children's mental health services from its roots dating back to the end of the 19th century with the opening of court and community clinic services, such as the Institute of Juvenile Research and Judge Baker clinics. These initiatives and the subsequent child guidance movement (supported in the 1920s through the Commonwealth Fund) were manifestations of that era's interest in progressive social intervention for children and their families. Subsequent decades (1930s–1950s) witnessed further progress and gains in the field with the gradual development of child psychiatry as a clinical and academic discipline, culminating in the founding of the American Academy of Child & Adolescent Psychiatry in 1954. Since then, the field of child psychiatry has continued to be influenced by significant advances in science, changes in care standards and practices, an evolving marketplace, and changing public perceptions of mental illness/health.

The Federal Role

Federal focus on mental health was scant in the first half of the century, with core responsibilities for mentally ill individuals of all ages residing with states and local communities. The passage of the Community Mental Health Center Construction Act (CMHC) in 1963 began to change this, although progress was slow. As described in the report *Crisis in Child Mental Health*, published 7 years later by the Joint Commission on Mental Health of Children, little national attention or resource was dedicated to the needs of children and their families at that time.

In 1972, the CMHC Act was extended, with the responsibilities of community mental health centers expanded to include services for children. Again, however, funding was limited for communities to implement programming. The President's Commission on Mental Health (1978) helped children and adolescents with severe emotional disturbances become designated as a priority service population. Finally in the 1980s, under the Alcohol, Drug Abuse, and Mental Health Block Grant program, joint federal and state funding was instituted, with a formula calling for 25% of funding to be dedicated to children and adolescents.[10]

Evolution of the Service Array

This allocation of funding set the stage because it fostered development of dedicated services for children and adolescents. The concept of the mental health "continuum of care" began to arise, expanding the minimalist array of inpatient and outpatient care to include day and residential treatment programs along with case management services. During the 70s and 80s, the elaboration of more formal diagnostic systems (ie, the Diagnostic Standard Manual of the American Psychiatric Association) and the beginnings of the modern psychopharmacologic era fostered a trend toward the medicalization of services, with expansive growth in the use of hospital and residential treatment services. This occurred in both public and private arenas. Concomitantly, in other public child-serving agencies, interventionist strategies increased as courts, social welfare, and juvenile justice departments attended more actively to issues of child abuse, delinquency, and familial dysfunction, with concomitant greater use of out-of-home placement and increased attention to mental health treatment needs.

These trends created significant economic and programmatic pressures on service agencies and private insurers so that managed care strategies were elaborated to curtail access to and intensity of service delivery. Most particularly in the private sector, use of inpatient and intensive residential care was sharply curtailed, with restrictive admissions criteria and limited lengths of stay imposed. One consequence of these trends was a shift in cost for intensive services to the public sector, further enhancing pressures to contain out-of-home placement activities and costs.

Beyond these pressures, the emergence of more community-based and family-centered system approaches has been supported by (1) a decline in stigma and a greater acceptance of mental health treatment of mental illnesses, (2) the rise of the consumer and family advocacy movement, (3) a reappraisal of the cost–benefit analysis of institutional services for youth, (4) further advances in clinical psychopharmacologic, psychotherapeutic, and psychosocial treatment capacities, (5) an increased willingness of child-serving institutions to work collaboratively, (6) success in political advocacy and class action litigation activities, and (7) facilitative funding and eligibility under Medicaid's Early and Periodic Screening, Diagnostic, and Treatment program.

The consequences have been a progressive evolution in public policy to the current state of affairs, with mental health standards and practice now more systemically integrated with overall societal efforts on behalf of children and families.

Systems of Care (1980–Present)

Two seminal contributions define the formal beginning of the system of care movement. The first of these came from the application of social research findings to public policy deliberations regarding the needs of children and their families. The second was the incorporation of consumer-oriented and -driven principles as components of the federal agenda for mental health services.

The leader of the first effort was Jane Knitzer, EdD,[11] whose 1983 manuscript "Unclaimed Children: The Failure of Public Responsibility to Children and Adolescents in Need of Mental Health Services," sponsored by Children's Defense Fund, highlighted the dilemmas in then-current practice of referring large numbers of youth in state custody to residential care away from family and community.

Concurrently in the 1980s, the National Institute for Mental Health instituted the Child and Adolescent Service System Project (CASSP), which elucidated core guidelines, the CASSP Principles, that continue to form the bedrock of policy guidance for public sector mental health programming. These principles strongly supported the concept of providing mental health services in a social and ecologic context, focused on community-based support for families. These principles include the following:

Access to comprehensive service array
Individualized, least-restrictive care
Culturally and clinically competent services
Parent involvement, advocacy, and rights
Interagency, case-managed, coordinated, and collaborative services
Early identification and intervention
Transitions to adult services

Further elaboration of system of care principles came shortly after in 1986, with Stroul and Freidman's,[12] *A System of Care for Children and Youth with Severe Emotional Disturbances*, which detailed the characteristics and challenges of the evolving service model. Numerous demonstration projects were soon in place seeking to bring these principles into operational reality, including the Alaska Youth Demonstration Project (1980s); the Ventura Project (Ventura County, California, 1980s); Vermont's Wraparound project (1980s); the Fort Bragg Demonstration Project (1980s); and the eight Robert Wood Johnson/Mental Health Services Program for Youth sites (early 1990s).

System of care innovation was given further impetus by the Washington Business Group on Health under the leadership of Mary Jane England, MD and Bob Cole, PhD whose efforts focused on addressing the fiscal and organizational challenges that would need to be addressed in communities seeking to revamp their service arrays.[13]

The most definitive federal influence on system of care came in 1992 with the passage of the Children' Mental Health Initiative (CMHI) by the Comprehensive Community Mental Health Services for Children and Their Families program, which incorporated the CASSP Principles as core expectations for public sector systems.

Since that time, the Child, Adolescent, and Family Branch of SAMHSA's CMHS initiated a project of system of care grants that has continued to the present, with more than 144 sites now having been funded. These grants to states, counties, tribal groups, and territorial authorities encourage implementation of the CASSP Principles in local service systems. Included in the grant's priorities have been supports for social marketing, consumer organization development, advocacy, augmented services, outcomes research, and staff training. Service goals have supported family-driven, community-based service delivery with emphasis on consumer empowerment, cultural competence, use of mentoring and local supports, case management, and interagency coordination.

Included in the CMHI legislation was a requirement for evaluation at a national level to characterize the demographics of the service population, changes and change processes of evolving systems, clinical outcomes of services provided, levels of consumer satisfaction, costs and cost effectiveness of services, and, more recently, sustainability of system of care innovations.

The system of care model has been favorably noted in successive federal policy reviews, including the 1999 Report of the Surgeon General on Mental Health,[14] the 2003 New Freedom Commission on Mental Health report,[15] and SAMHSA's Federal Action Agenda in 2005.

SYSTEMS OF CARE IN OPERATION
Core Features of a System of Care

A simple but valuable expression of the goal of systems of care is to increase the number of children who are "in home, at school, out of trouble." To achieve these ends, systems of care endeavor to have the following characteristics:

   Clinical services are accessible and available in community settings, such as schools, youth centers, and homes.
   Services are organized as collaborative ventures with other child-serving agencies (eg, child welfare, probation, special education, developmental disability, health).
   Consumer empowerment and responsibility (family and youth "voice and choice") is reinforced with "strengths-based" approaches in treatment planning and service delivery. Care is congruent with family values and goals, merging wrap-around supports and services with traditional mental health interventions.
   Clinical outreach and case management are central elements of service delivery, seeking to match family needs and strengths with community-based supports. Paraprofessional mental health staff, without licensure, and community and family volunteers work as mentors with youth and their families, pursuant to individualized service plans and clinical oversight.
   Child psychiatric and other mental health professional involvement is supported to ensure needed clinical assessment and treatment interventions.

Local public health and human service agencies collaborate in integrating mental health services in their operational planning and funding considerations.

Consumer-directed Care

A central tenet of the system of care model has been to focus on organizing services around the needs of children and their families see **Box 1**. Therefore, public mental health and other child-serving agencies are being called on to help families in having primary decision-making roles in the care of their children and to support their voice in negotiations on the policies and procedures governing care for all children in their community. Enumerated principles of consumer-directed care include enabling access to information, fostering shared decision making, encouraging family owner-ship and responsibility for outcomes, providing access to peer support, assuring services that are culturally and linguistically appropriate, shifting from provider- to family-driven models, and supporting training to advance consumer-centric policy and practices.[16]

Family advocacy has been a core feature of the federally funded programs, reflect-ing the reality that families can have significant local political influence to advance the implementation of consumer-centric care. The Federation of Families for Children's Mental Health and its subsidiary, Youth M.O.V.E., have joined traditional advocacy organizations such as the National Alliance on Mental Illness, and Mental Health America in supporting systems that provide consumer-directed care. These advocacy organizations have had considerable influence on local, state, and national policy discussions.

Wraparound

The embodiment of consumer-directed care in children's mental health is the wrap-around process, which is emerging as an evidence-based methodology to serve chil-dren who have complex needs in the context of and with the support of their families.

The fundamental goal involves empowering families to build on strengths and capacities to overcome challenges to the adaptive well-being of their children so

---

Box 1
Web resources

National Federation of Families for Children's Mental Health: http://www.ffcmh.org

Institute for Family-Centered Care: http://www.familycenteredcare.org

Family Voices: http://www.familyvoices.org

PACERCenter (Parent Advocacy Coalition for Educational Rights): http://www.PACER.org

Youth M.O.V.E.: http://www.youthmove.us

American Academy of Child & Adolescent Psychiatry: http://www.aacap.org

National Wraparound Initiative: http://www.rtc.pdx.edu/nwi

National Wraparound Initiative/About Wraparound: http://www.rtc.pdx.edu/nwi/aboutwraparound.php

PaperBoat: http://www.paperboat.com

Children and Adults with Attention Deficit/Hyperactivity Disorder: http://www.chadd.org

Mental Health American: http://www.nmha.org

National Alliance on Mental Illness: http://www.nami.org

they can achieve greater self-sufficiency. Wraparound entails a collaborative team-based approach to service and support planning to foster engagement, ownership, and responsibility by youth and family in partnership with involved providers, agency staff, and other system stakeholders.[17]

A system of care's fidelity to the precepts of wraparound process can be measured by the Wraparound Fidelity Index (WFI), which assesses the following phases of treatment: engagement/team preparation; plan development; implementation; and transition. The WFI enumerates specific skill sets and service characteristics for each phase. Criteria derived from the CASSP Principles (eg, family-driven, team-based, collaborative, community-based, culturally competent, individualized, strengths-based, natural supports, unconditional, and outcome-based) provide guides for evaluation. High-fidelity wraparound is compatible with and encourages combining professional services with community-based supports.[18]

Paradigm Shift

The apparent paradox of having families who are struggling in their care for their children having leadership roles in treatment processes and policy development is a challenge to traditional provider-centric orientations that frame decision making as originating with and based on the provider's professional expertise.

The new model requires that clinical understanding of a case be fully rooted in the context of the youth/family's lived experience, defined by family and as evidenced in the family's culture and life history. It thus requires a process of "strengths and culture" discovery as pivotal in assessment, planning, and intervention phases of the clinical process. This effort seeks to ensure that treatment services and supports chosen are provided to optimally suit the family's objectives and maximize collaboration toward the desired goals.

For CAPs working in the public mental health sector, this means a need to expand on the traditional skills set of evaluation, diagnosis, and treatment to include participation with a broadened interdisciplinary team process that highlights youth/family prerogatives and responsibilities, and expands the scope of clinical interventions beyond the clinic office into the real world of patients and their families. Family-centered practice, of course, does not undo the clinician's role or authority, particularly in the area of safety and medical expertise, but it does require a reframing of the relationship with the patient and family toward a collaborative orientation with all stakeholders in their system of care.

The Institute of Medicine's (IOM) "new rules" for a 21st Century Health Care System[19] are in concert with the system of care model, with enunciated principles of care that state:

Care is based on continuous healing relationships
Care is customized according to needs and values
The patient is the source of control
Knowledge is shared and information flows freely
Transparency is necessary

For children's mental health, the IOM "new rules" encourage a focus on healing relationships within families in the community; elucidating and addressing individual and family needs, values, and strengths; placing control and responsibility in the hands of youth and their families; and sharing knowledge transparently in support of optimal decision making by the youth and family, in concert with the supporting treatment team.

Box 2
System-based practice competencies in child and adolescent psychiatry

Knowledge of core clinical competencies in psychiatry, including

- Biopsychosocial perspective
- Developmental approach
- The dynamics of healing relationships
- Family systems theory
- Recovery and resiliency models
- Case management process
- Community resources, including other child-serving agency systems
- Advocacy and outreach techniques
- Leadership styles and responsibilities
- Funding sources and eligibility
- Wraparound approaches and system of care program design elements

Skills in the application of clinical and scientific knowledge to

- Act as a medical officer
- Identify and address safety considerations
- Perform diagnostic assessments, formulate intervention plans, conduct treatment
- Conduct psychotherapy (individual, family, group)
- Manage psychopharmacologic interventions
- Communicate with respect and in context of privacy expectations
- Collaborate with stakeholders within the family and among agencies with cultural and linguistic competency
- Use a strengths and culture discovery process
- Normalize the recovery process and address service transitions
- Advocate for in-need populations and individuals in need
- Participate and support wraparound

Attitudes of interest and investment in

- Applying mental health expertise to complex psychosocial domains
- Consumer-driven care
- Encouraging and enhancing youth "voice and choice" and family leadership
- Multidisciplinary treatment and interagency collaboration
- Clinical supervision and oversight of staff providing non-traditional service and supports
- Providing in-home and in-community care
- Wraparound approaches
- Advancing public health goals and evaluating outcomes
- Optimizing cost effective approaches

CHILD PSYCHIATRIC COMPETENCY IN SYSTEM OF CARE PRACTICE

The emerging and expanding system of care model presents a challenge to established practitioners and early career and trainee child/adolescent psychiatrists (and their educators) for whom great needs but limited resources exist for relevant medical education. System-based practice is one of the core areas of proficiency prescribed by the Accreditation Council on Graduate Medical Education (ACGME) in its oversight of all residency training programs.[20]

For child psychiatrists the system of care model is a key element of system-based practice competency. As more fully enumerated in the systems-based practice in child & adolescent psychiatry—a resource guide for training and clinical care, under development by the American Academy of Child and Adolescent Psychiatry's Work Group on Community-Based Systems of Care,[21] competency is measured by a CAP showing the knowledge, skills, and attitudes as listed in **Box 2**.

CAPs have great potential to expand their roles as key participants in systems of care, with opportunities that include being a clinician, consultant, catalyst, collaborator, advocate, and administrator. CAPs competent in systems-based practice have exceptional professional opportunities to serve children and youth with multidimensional and multisystem problems, to support innovation in service design and delivery, to act as a consultant and provider with social agency programs, to work with family organizations, to address disparities in health care delivery, to pursue cost effectiveness and improved outcomes, and to advocate for mental health informed policy.

SUMMARY

Although the future of the systems of care model continues to evolve, the core values of child psychiatry are clearly well supported and can be well served in this emerging arena of public children's mental health service delivery. A substantial body of evidence supports the concepts and practices of family-driven care congruent with wraparound principles and practices. Individual and system outcomes data show efficacy for programs that integrate traditional professional services with consumer-centric wraparound approaches, such as mentoring, team decision making, and community-based services and supports. Integrative interagency practice, fostering cross-agency collaboration and funding to address the needs of at-risk population, has been shown to be central in providing supports for families and youth. Federal support of the CASSP Principles as guides for system development has an important role, as does consumer and professional advocacy to improve public mental health services. **Box 1** provides a list of Web resources.

ACKNOWLEDGMENTS

The author wishes to acknowledge the support of the members of the Work Group on Community Systems of Care of the American Academy of Child & Adolescent Psychiatry for their contributions to the field and to key reference resources noted in the bibliography. Special thanks to Kaye McGinty, MD, Mary Grealish, MEd, and Brigitte Manteuffel, PhD for their contributions.

REFERENCES

1. Pumariega A, Winters N, editors. Part one: conceptual foundations of systems of care. The handbook of child and adolescent systems of care: the new community psychiatry. San Francisco (CA): Jossey-Bass; 2003.

2. AACAP. Practice parameter on child and adolescent mental health care in community systems of care. J Am Acad Child Adolesc Psychiatry 2007;46:284–99.

3. Annual Report to Congress on the Evaluation of the Comprehensive Community Mental Health Services for Children and Their Families Program (2001). Available at: http://mentalhealth.samhsa.gov/publications/allpubs/CB-E201/default.asp. Accessed August 15, 2009.

4. Osher TA, Osher D. The paradigm shift to true collaboration with families. J Child Fam Stud 2002;11:47–60.

5. Winters NA, Metz WP. The wraparound approach in systems of care. Psychiatr Clin North Am 2009;32(1):135–51.

6. Chenven M, Brady B. Collaboration across disciplines among agencies within systems of care. In: Pumariega A, Winters N, editors. The handbook of child and adolescent systems of care: the new community psychiatry. San Francisco (CA): Jossey-Bass; 2003. p. 66–81.

7. Hernandez M, Hodges S. Applying a theory of change approach to interagency planning in child mental health. Am J Community Psychol 2006;38:165–75.

8. SAMHSA National Mental Health information Center, Center for Mental Health Services; Child, Adolescent and Family Branch, program summaries, annual reports to Congress. Available at: http://mentalhealth.samhsa.gov/cmhs/ChildrensCampaign/about.asp. Accessed September 18, 2009.

9. Manteuffel B, Stephens RL, Brashears F, et al. Evaluation results and systems of care: a review. In: Stroul BA, Blau BA, editors. The system of care handbook: transforming mental health services for children, youth, and families. Baltimore (MD): Paul H. Brookes Publishing Co., Inc; 2008. p. 25–69.

10. Lourie IS, Katz-Leavey J, DeCarolis G, et al. The role of the federal government. In: Stroul BA, editor. Children's mental health: creating systems of care in a changing society. Baltimore (MD): Brooks Publishing; 1996. p. 99–114.

11. Knitzer J. Unclaimed children: the failure of public responsibility to children and adolescents in need of mental health services. Washington, DC: Children's Defense Fund; 1983.

12. Stroul BA, Freidman RA. A system of care for children and youth with severe emotional disturbances (Rev ed.), Washington, DC: Georgetown University Child Development Center, National Technical Assistance Center for Child Mental Health; 1994.

13. Cole RF, Poe S, Partnerships for care: systems of care for children with serious emotional disturbances and their families. Washington, DC: Washington Business Group on Health; 1993.

14. U.S. Public Health Service. Office of the surgeon general, mental health: a report of the surgeon general. Rockville (MD): US Department of Health and Human Services; 1999.

15. Hogan M, Hefferman C, Eichenaver H, et al. New freedom commission on mental health, achieving the Promise: transforming mental health care in America. Executive summary Pub. No. SMA-03-3831. Rockville (MD): DHHS; 2003. Available at: www.mentalhealthcommission.gov. Accessed September 18, 2009.

16. Osher TA, Blau GM, Osher DM. Shifting gears: a curriculum guide to family driven care [CD]. Rockville (MD): Federal of Families for Children's Mental Health; 2006.

17. Walker J. How, and why, does wraparound work: a theory of change. Portland (OR): National Wraparound Initiative, Portland State University; 2008.

18. National Wraparound Initiative. Available at: http://www.rtc.pdx.edu/nwi/aboutwraparound.php. Accessed August 15, 2009.

19. Institute of Medicine. Formulating new rules to redesign and improve care, in crossing the quality chasm: a new health system for the 21st century. Washington, DC: National Academy Press; 2001. 61–89.
20. Accreditation Council of Graduate Medical Education. Program requirement for residency education in child and adolescent psychiatry. Available at: http://www/acgme.org/acWebstie/downloads/RRC_progReq/405pr07012007.pdf. Accessed August 15, 2009.
21. McGinty K, Chenven M, Winters N, et al. American Academy of Child and Adolescent Psychiatry work group on systems of care, systems-based practice. Child and adolescent psychiatry—A resource guide for training and clinical care [draft]. Washington, DC: AACAP; 2009.

Index

Note: Page numbers of article titles are in **boldface** type.

Child Adolesc Psychiatric Clin N Am 19 (2010) 175–182
doi:10.1016/S1056-4993(09)00110-2
1056-4993/09/$ – see front matter © 2010 Elsevier Inc. All rights reserved.
childpsych.theclinics.com

Moving?

Make sure your subscription moves with you!

To notify us of your new address, find your **Clinics Account Number** (located on your mailing label above your name), and contact customer service at:

Email: journalscustomerservice-usa@elsevier.com

800-654-2452 (subscribers in the U.S. & Canada)
314-447-8871 (subscribers outside of the U.S. & Canada)

Fax number: 314-447-8029

Elsevier Health Sciences Division
Subscription Customer Service
3251 Riverport Lane
Maryland Heights, MO 63043

*To ensure uninterrupted delivery of your subscription, please notify us at least 4 weeks in advance of move.

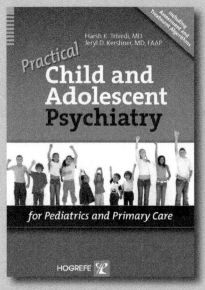
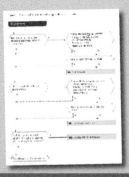
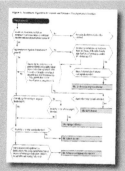
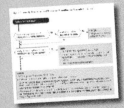

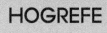

Printed and bound by CPI Group (UK) Ltd, Croydon, CR0 4YY

03/10/2024

01040441-0019